The Yogi Entrepreneur

A Guide to Earning a Mindful Living Through Yoga

By Darren Main

D1367780

Printed and bound in the USA

Cover Design & Author Photo by Jasper Trout
http://troutfarmphotodesign.com

Typesetting, ebook & Print Production by Michael Fantasia
www.linkedin.com/in/mfantasia

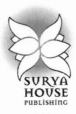

SURYA
HOUSE
PUBLISHING

Surya Rising Books
PO Box 14584
San Francisco, CA 94114

Trademarks and Disclaimer

Dedication

Arthur Leiper*

You saw potential in me long before I could see it in myself. Although you never stood on your head, or did a downward dog, you taught me the most important things I know about teaching yoga and your inspiration passes through me every day.

*See appendix for more on the life of Arthur Leiper.

Endorsements

When I read *Yogi Entrepreneur*, I was struck not only by Darren Main's thoughtfulness about the topic and his experience in the field, but also by the personal and very real way he conveyed his information. It was more like having a very useful and interesting conversation with a wise and funny friend rather than reading a "how to" book.

It's too bad that we all didn't have this book when we began to find our way as yoga teachers. It would have made that first part of the journey easier and much more enjoyable. Highly recommended for both beginning and experienced teachers.
—Judith Hanson Lasater, Ph.D., PT,
   Yoga teacher since 1971, and author of eight books, including *Yogabody* and *What We Say Matters*.
   www.judithlasater.com

Finally, a much needed book on the business art of yoga. Many of us have the skills and wisdom of yoga to proficiently reach out to people as teachers. Managing the business end of yoga is our downfall. Highly skilled and extraordinary yoga teachers whose career's are shining successes ultimately fail due lack of business skills. This book is a powerful guide to facilitate what teachers are qualified to offer and at the same time make a successful living for themselves.

Darren speaks from his own successful experience and journey in yoga. His insights are highly informative for those who find the business side of yoga more stressful than successful.
—Yogi Amrit Desai
   Founder of Kripalu Yoga and author of *Amrit Yoga*
   www.amrityoga.org

Yoga and business can be perceived as oxymoronic. For the yoga teacher looking to make a career of doing what they love, Darren Main's book, *The Yogi Entrepreneur*, is invaluable. We will highly recommend it to our teachers and those in our Teacher Training programs.
—Trevor Tice
   Founder CorePower Yoga
   www.corepoweryoga.com

Darren Main has done it again with *The Yogi Entrepreneur*. His in-depth analysis and advice offer unique insight that you won't find in yoga manuals. This masterful book, like his second book *Yoga and the Path of the Urban Mystic* should be required reading in all teacher training courses. This masterful work covers every angle of becoming a successful yoga entrepreneur from how to begin, to branding, accounting, and inspiring others. The personal reflections take the reader deep into the ethics and principles of yoga in a way that is unsurpassed.
—Darren Littlejohn, RYT,
    Author of the 12-Step Buddhist
    www.the12stepbuddhist.com

Yoga teacher Darren Main eloquently describes how the business of yoga is more than the time spent teaching on a mat. Yoga is a way of life, but the business of yoga requires a practical blueprint if one wishes to succeed. Main's newest book, *The Yogi Entrepreneur*, gives the reader the critical principals that will allow for their careers to thrive. Informative and insightful, *The Yogi Entrepreneur* is essential reading for anyone who desires to teach yoga as a profession.
—Jeffrey Small
    author of THE BREATH OF GOD
    www.jeffreysmall.com

Darren's done it again! He makes tough topics such as yoga philosophy and the business of yoga accessible to all. This is a must-read for yoga teachers, aspiring teachers, and mindful entrepreneurs looking to make a difference in the world through their work. A great tool for the yoga community and beyond.
—Kimberly Wilson
    author of *Hip Tranquil Chick* and *Tranquilista*
    founder of Tranquil Space Yoga, Washington, DC
    Designer of TranquiliT Clothing
    www.kimberlywilson.com

In today's yoga world there is little offered in the way of conducting your yoga business. Even more, there is little offered in how to do this ethically. Darren Main not only offers a powerful path in how to thrive in

the "Yoga Business" world, but how to do it without losing "your yoga." Congratulations to Darren in pioneering and paving this path for the yoga community.
—Aaron Star
   Founder of Blue Osa Spa, Costa Rica
   www.blueosa.com

Whether you teach yoga full-time or part-time, this is your ultimate go-to resource for understanding the business of yoga. As a part-time yoga teacher in Washington, DC, one of my biggest fears of transitioning into teaching full time is not being able to effectively run my own yoga business. Darren guides you through responsible accounting and innovative marketing while he shares his secrets to his own success by providing simple, yet direct guidance to help turn your calling into a reality and to stand out in an ever increasing pool of yoga teachers.
—Marshall Sanders
   Yoga Instructor, Washington, DC
   www.yogimarshall.com

The Yogi Entrepreneur is the how-to book that so many teachers have been seeking. By exploring essential topics like continuing education, teacher ethics, and mindful marketing, Darren Man has written a much-needed guidebook for new and seasoned teachers alike. This book will be required reading in Yoga Tree teacher trainings, and our entire teaching staff will be encouraged to read and reread it with a highlighter in hand!
—Tara Dale
   Director of Yoga Tree, San Francisco
   www.yogatreesf.com

I mentor dozens of new teachers every year and Darren's clear cut directions and simplified approach to meaningful and mindful earnings is a great reminder to me, and a useful guide for everyone, to remain conscious in everything we do. We can live a life filled with passion and earn a living that deepens our respect of self and of others on this amazing path.
—Les Leventhal
   International Yoga Teacher
   www.YogaWithLes.com

With this book, Darren provides a much-needed resource for the modern Yogi, in a world where bookkeeper, advertising agent, and yoga teacher seldom appear in the same sentence. His years of experience bring great depth and insight into the forgotten, but so important side of establishing yoga as a viable and sustainable business that can continue to grow and bring wealth, health, and happiness to our culture.

—Michael Watson

Michael Watson

Founder of *Mindful Integration*

Director of *Bermuda Integrative Health Coop ltd*
www.mindfulintegration.com
www.healthcoop.net

I can't think of a better, more qualified person to speak with authority about making a living in the mystic arts than Darren Main.

—Dr. Jallen Rix

Sexologist and author of *Ex-Gay No Way: Survival and Recovery from Religious Abuse*
www.doctorrix.com

Everyone who's ever taken a shower has an idea. It's the person who gets out of the shower, dries off and does something about it who makes a difference. —*Nolan Bushnell*

CONTENTS

INTRODUCTION

Are you bored with life? Then throw yourself into some work you believe in with all your heart; live for it, die for it, and you will find happiness that you had thought could never be yours.—Dale Carnegie

The Decision to Teach

When my sister Jennifer was a little girl she would run around the back yard in her bathing suit sporting tinfoil bracelets, a makeshift tiara, and a length of twine hanging from her waist. Her dream when she grew up was to be Wonder Woman—her goal to rid the world of monsters. A noble goal to be sure, but as she started school, any notion of taking on the evils of the world was quickly replaced by the near-constant message that in order to be successful in this world you needed to find an occupation that pays the rent and has good health care benefits. Unfortunately for my sister and for many other would-be heroes and heroines, being a superhero doesn't come with a pension. So more practical occupations were pursued until one day, we woke up and discovered that this occupational pragmatism had become our kryptonite.

Yet for some of us, that desire to heal the world remains strong, though buried under layers of so-called responsibility. And when that inner hero begins to wake up, we realize that we are called to do something unconventional. After years of striving to become 'responsible' we come to realize that our inner hero has fallen into a deep sleep—our jobs may have provided ample food for our bellies, but our spirits are gaunt.

While teaching yoga may not be as glamorous as crime fighting in spandex, it is a powerful medicine in this world. But like any super hero we need to take on two roles if we want to be really effective. Wonder Woman needed Diana Prince, Batman needed Bruce Wayne, and Spider-Man needed Peter Parker. Likewise, yoga teachers also need to be entrepreneurs.

Like most young people, I didn't plan to teach yoga when I was in grade school. As a boy I dreamed of being a fireman or an astronaut, not a yoga teacher. Even through most of my college years, I looked toward the more practical and responsible occupation of social work.

My own yogic journey was born out of the Twelve Steps. At the age of seventeen, I hit an emotional and spiritual bottom, due in large part to drug abuse. It took a number of failed attempts at sobriety and a suicide attempt before I really took my recovery seriously. However, once I did have my awakening, it became clear to me that I wanted to devote my life to helping others find a better way to live.

Following high school I enrolled in college with a major in social work and a minor in psychology and counseling. During this time, I had begun a yoga practice to support my recovery. From the first class I felt like I had come home. I knew yoga was such a wonderful and healing tool for me, but coming to terms with the fact that I, the screwed up teenager who was just struggling to stay sober, could actually teach, was not something I could even fathom in the beginning.

In time, however, I became increasingly unsatisfied with my duties as a social worker. I had not even graduated from college and I was already starting to see the limits of the profession. This is not to say that I don't have tremendous respect for social work and the hard-working and dedicated professionals who look out for others. I was simply feeling a tug from deep within calling me to share my passion for yoga.

So in my third year of school, I dropped out to spend more time in an ashram where I could study yoga more intensely and become certified to teach others. Following my heart was an incredibly liberating experience, although I was not yet sure how I could make a living teaching yoga.

Back then, things were much different. If you had a weekly class with ten students, you were like a rock star in the yoga world. The demographics were also quite different. In my first yoga class, I was by far the youngest person in the room; most people were in their thirties and forties. I was also the only man in the class. Today, millions of people are practicing yoga in one form or another every day. People of every demographic are practicing, and my average class size is between forty and sixty people.

The Business of Yoga

One of the things I realized from the start was that if I was going to devote my life to teaching yoga, I would need to treat it like a real business—a mindful business to be sure, but a business nonetheless. The problem was, like most yoga teachers, I was more interested in teaching handstands than hanging flyers, and I was more interested in meditation than balancing my checkbook.

Learning to be a businessman was not something that came naturally to me. I felt a conflict within me about being a spiritual teacher who was also business savvy. What I have come to realize, however, is that by treating my work as a yoga teacher like a mindful business, I have the ability to reach out to more people, while at the same time supporting myself in a way that is both ethical and beneficial to society.

This book is the culmination of many years of struggling with the business side of teaching yoga. My hope is that it will help you to organize your thoughts and develop a career that offers the amazing practice of yoga to many people in your community. Our world is so hungry for spiritual awareness, and your decision to teach others this ancient practice is such a gift. I sincerely hope this book will help you become more effective in sharing that gift.

About This Book

This book is divided into three parts. Part One deals with the process of becoming a teacher, beginning with your decision about what kind of teacher you would like to be, and moving on to choosing a program that best suits your goals, your budget, and your schedule.

In Part Two we will explore the business of teaching yoga. We will learn the ins and outs of working for yourself as a yoga teacher, from finding a job, to professional ethics, and leading workshops and retreats.

Part Three will deal with marketing, and I will offer dozens of free and low cost marketing techniques to help you spread the word about your teaching. I will also provide some guidance on developing your own website.

This book, of course, is not the final word on running your unique business, but I do hope it will help you organize your thoughts and mine the depths of your creativity to begin a professional, ethical, and rewarding career as a yoga teacher. Most of all, I hope you will find the tools you need to reach out to the people in your community who are looking for yoga, and have been waiting for the right teacher to come along to help them find healing, wholeness, and spiritual renewal.

Namaste,

Darren Main

www.darrenmain.com

Part One:
Becoming a Teacher

Everyone has his own specific vocation or mission in life; everyone must carry out a concrete assignment that demands fulfillment. Therein he cannot be replaced, nor can his life be repeated; thus, everyone's task is as unique as his specific opportunity to implement it.
—Viktor E. Frankl

CHAPTER 1:
SHARING YOUR PRACTICE

*Your calling refers to a personal interest, attraction, inclination, drive,
or passion that is usually (but not always) of a higher order. It isn't
just something you want to do, but rather something you need to do,
something that captures your imagination, touches you deeply and
absorbs you, whether or not you can explain why.*
—*Dan Millman*, THE FOUR PURPOSES OF LIFE

For many years now I have been leading yoga teacher training programs,
and in that role I have seen thousands of people become certified to teach.
It's always interesting for me to watch people after graduation.

Some people go on to become very successful with a sizable following,
while others never really develop as teachers. In more conventional career
choices, the really successful people in any given field tend to be the ones
who study hard, have a plan after they complete their schooling, and keep
their eye on the ball. All this is true for yoga teachers as well, and it's what
much of this book is about. However, teaching yoga is much more than
knowing your alignment and having flashy business cards.

Teaching yoga requires passion for the practice and absent that, no amount
of marketing and training will make you a success. One of the most
successful teachers in San Francisco, Janet Stone [www.janetstoneyoga.com],
has a huge following of students. She teaches a vigorous and sweaty class,
while also blending in chanting and a great sense of community. Her classes
often have more than one hundred students in attendance. Clearly she is
doing something right.

Unfortunately for many other yoga teachers who want to experience her
level of success, that goal seems very evasive. There are more teachers in
San Francisco than I can count who try to copy Janet's formula, and can't
understand why their classes don't draw the huge crowds that Janet's do.

What they fail to realize about Janet is that her class is much more than a collection of techniques that she employs. It is much more than making people sweat or leading some chanting. In other words, her classes are much greater than the sum of the parts because the glue that holds them together is Janet's enthusiasm for her own practice and her willingness to share that practice with others. Janet's teaching and practice are unique to her and no one can copy or emulate that with any degree of success.

I have another friend, Jennifer Gray, who teaches classes and workshops at her studio, The Yoga Center of Minneapolis [www.yogacentermpls. com]. Jennifer had struggled her whole life with her weight and body image. She had tried every diet and weight loss technique she could find, with no lasting results. Exercise was also a problem for her because she felt uncomfortable at the gym.

When she found yoga, she was able to start feeling good about herself and her body. Out of that improved sense of self, her diet naturally changed, and she was able to lose weight and keep it off. This gave her a natural passion for yoga and she decided to become a teacher. It was out of this passion that her "Big-Ass Yoga" program was developed. Now she works extensively with other women who are struggling with their body image issues, and she is having great success.

In addition to being a skilled teacher, Jennifer brings something that few other teachers can bring to the table—her challenges and successes in dealing with her weight and body image. Her students can identify with her and she inspires them to keep coming back, even when things get tough, because she lives her yoga and they can see the fruits of her labors.

Jennifer and Janet seemingly have little in common. Their teaching styles and their life stories are not closely related. However, they both have a passion for their yoga practice, and out of that, their success as teachers is born. If either of them were to do it just for the money or try to teach the other's class, they would no doubt fall flat, but because their own personal practice has brought them healing, others who identify with them flock to their classes.

Yoga is all the rage right now, and I'm sure many people look at the yoga industry and see only dollar signs. Certainly there is money to be made, but that money and success will never come by trying to sell people yoga in the same way a car salesman might push his wares. Success comes from standing in your truth. If you feel drawn to teach gentle classes, there will be students out there who will be drawn to you. If you feel drawn to teach more athletic yoga, there will be students who will want what you have to offer. Maybe you want to focus on the spiritual, the stress management, or the healing aspects of yoga. Whichever you choose, there will be students who will be interested in what you have to offer.

The key is to know what you love and then offer it to the world. This is the first step to becoming a successful yoga teacher, and the importance of this step cannot be overstated. Everything else we will be exploring from this point forward will be determined by your taking this step in the most honest, open, and effective way possible. To proceed without really considering the teacher you want to be, is to spend a lot of time on wasted endeavors and to reap more disappointment than success.

My father, a farmer, once told me that animals can sense fear. When we were helping him feed the animals on the farm, he taught my brother, sister, and me to remain calm or the animals would get spooked. Yoga students have a similar skill. They can sense a phony a mile away. If you are not authentic in sharing your practice with them, they will know it. If you are attempting to teach them only what you think is trendy and popular, for money or ego, they will instinctively know and will avoid your classes.

Personal Reflections and Journaling

Throughout this book I will be offering some questions on various topics. These questions do not have right or wrong answers. They are simply designed for your own personal reflection. In order to really grow as a teacher and as a business person, it is essential that you search your soul for the most honest options possible, and then carefully consider your answers.

My strong suggestion is that you keep a journal and write about each question as truthfully as you can. Again, this is not about getting the right answers—it's about reflecting on the teacher you want to be, the students you want to work with, and the best way you can reach out to those students in ways that are both creative and in keeping with yogic ethics (Yamas and Niyamas).

The more time you take with this process, the more effective this book will be in helping you achieve your goals. I will offer you a number of tips and resources, but in truth, none of them will be useful if you are not internally clear about the yoga business you want to grow. Taking the time to journal will serve to order your thoughts and bring clarity of purpose to your business plan.

Personal Reflections

◊ What type of yoga do I feel most drawn to teach?
(Iyengar, Anusara, Ashtanga, Restorative, Flow, etc.)

◊ In addition to poses and breathing techniques, what other elements
do I want in my class? (i.e., mediation, chanting, philosophy, etc.)

◊ How has my personal healing and growth influenced this decision?

◊ Which teachers do I admire and why?

◊ How will my teaching be similar to theirs?

◊ How will it be different?

◊ What teachers and styles of yoga have not interested me?

◊ What elements of those teaching styles were distracting, uninspiring
or discouraging for me?

◊ What unique qualities do I bring to my teaching?

◊ What types of people would benefit from my teaching style?

◊ What types of people might be better served by studying
with another teacher?

◊ Do I identify with any group, community or subculture to which I
could reach out? (i.e., Latino, queer, cancer survivors, Jewish, etc.)

◊ Do I have skills beyond teaching yoga that might make my
teaching more accessible to a specific group? (i.e., Fluent in a
foreign language, trained as a nurse, did social work, experience
working with children, etc.)

◊ What qualities do I have that make my voice unique in the
yoga community?

◊ How might those qualities attract students and make them feel
welcome in my class?

CHAPTER 2:
CHOOSING A TEACHER TRAINING PROGRAM

*Be the living expression of God's kindness. Kindness in your
face; Kindness in your eyes; Kindness in your smile; Let no one ever
come to you without leaving better and happier. —Mother Teresa*

Once you have decided what you want to offer, you will want to make sure
you have the best training possible to achieve your goals. If you are already
certified to teach, you will want to look at the many continuing education
options. If you have not yet completed a teacher certification, you have
some very important choices to make.

Let's look at your options and consider which will be best for you.
Please refer to the questions you answered in the last chapter to be clear
about your needs.

The Yoga Alliance
Because no legal guidelines currently exist for teaching yoga, *The Yoga
Alliance* [www.yogaalliance.org] was formed by a diverse board of
yoga professionals. Among its many functions, *The Yoga Alliance* has
composed minimum educational standards for yoga teachers and yoga
teacher training programs. Compliance with these broadly accepted
standards is an important credential to look for when choosing a
teacher training program. Since there are so many teacher training
programs out there, many gyms and yoga studios will not hire a teacher
who is not certified by the Alliance.

*Work performed with the right attitude is worship in action.
When you learn to work with love, your life will be an expression of joy.
—Yogi Amrit Desai*

Four Types of Training

There are more teacher training programs out there than I can possibly begin to list here; however, they generally fit into one of the following categories.

Category One: The Intensive

There are numerous intensives out there that are less than two hundred hours in length and focus on certain aspects of yoga rather than giving a full and well-rounded education. While I don't recommend these shorter programs for people who want to teach, they can be useful in helping you to deepen your own practice and to help you decide if you want to take your education to the next level. It is important to note that these shorter programs are not recognized by *The Yoga Alliance* and other professional organizations, so you will not be certified. Consequently, most gyms, health clubs, and yoga studios will not hire you with such limited training.

Category Two: The Weekend Warrior

The vast majority of training programs are 200 hours in length and cover a wide range of topics including alignment, teaching methodology, philosophy, anatomy, and other important topics that are essential to become a yoga teacher. Most of these programs model their curriculum after the guidelines set forth by *The Yoga Alliance*.

200-hour certifications generally come in two types. The first I call the weekend-warrior. In these programs you continue your daily life and attend teacher training classes and workshops on the weekends or in the evenings. Most programs last about four to six months. One of the nice qualities about Weekend Warrior programs is that you can continue with your life, and you don't need to place work responsibilities on hold.

The main drawback to the Weekend Warrior approach is that training to become a yoga teacher is intense. You will be studying a lot of anatomy, philosophy, alignment, and advanced yogic practices. Additionally, you will be required to maintain a regular yoga practice. All of this adds up to very little free time for family and friends and little precious leisure time.

The program I run at Yoga Tree in San Francisco [www.yogatreesf.org] falls into the Weekend Warrior category. The program is six months in length and we meet on Friday nights for two hours, and Saturdays and Sundays for three hours each. In addition to that, students are required to practice yoga six hours per week. Needless to say, this doesn't bode well for their social lives. It does, however, allow a lot of people to train to become teachers who would not otherwise be able to do so.

Category Three: The Dorm Room Style

The third type of teacher training is what I call the dorm room style, because it involves an extended stay. In this type of training you pack your bags and head to an ashram or retreat center for an extended period of time. Most are about one month long although some programs break up the training into two segments.

In order to fit 200 hours of training into such a short amount of time, dorm room style programs usually start early in the morning and conduct classes and workshops throughout the day breaking only for meals. The benefit of such programs is that you completely immerse yourself in the practice. By removing yourself from your life, the training closely resembles how the practice was taught in the ashrams of India and you are able to go deeply into the practice of yoga. The downside is that many people cannot take a month off from their lives. The cost of lodging and meals can also add to the overall cost of the program.

Category Four: 500-Hour Certifications

While the vast majority of programs are 200 hours in length, some are 500 hours or more. There are two different approaches to 500-hour certifications. The most common requires that you have a 200-hour certification under your belt as a pre-requisite and then offers a 300-hour program to bring your total to 500 hours. Many of these programs can be done as a continuation of a 200-hour program at a given school, but many schools will also recognize 200 hours from another school accredited by *The Yoga Alliance*.

There are programs that offer 500-hour trainings in one lump sum as well. These programs mostly hale from the Iyengar tradition and usually span the course of two years. The upside to these trainings is the extent of the information given. A lot can be learned with an additional three hundred hours. The downside is the financial and time commitment involved in 500-hour programs, which is considerably more, and can therefore be prohibitive for some people.

Continuing Education

Once you receive your basic certification it is important to continue to grow as a teacher and as a student. Perhaps you want to specialize in a certain area of yoga such as "core work," pranayama, or meditation. Maybe you want to work with children, seniors, or with cancer patients. Maybe you just want to brush up on your anatomy, Sanskrit, or alignment.

There are hundreds of courses out there to help you do all of this. Some of them are geared to a more general audience, while other workshops and trainings are reserved for existing teachers. Whatever the case, continuing your education is exceedingly important. To maintain your membership with *The Yoga Alliance*, you are required to do continuing education with a qualified teacher and report your continuing education hours to *The Yoga Alliance* on a regular basis.

How to Choose a Training Program

There are training programs all over the world representing every style of yoga imaginable. Trying to decide which one can be daunting, so considering the following five points may help you narrow it down.

Style

There is no point in taking a training that focuses on flow yoga if you only want to teach restorative yoga, or studying Iyengar yoga if you really want to teach Anusara yoga. Find a program that reflects what you want to teach.

Timing

Consider your own timing needs. If there is no way you can take a month off work, then there is no point in looking at programs that require that. Likewise, if you are a school-teacher and have summers free, a month-long program at a quiet ashram may be just the right fit.

Cost

The cost of various teacher-training programs can range quite a bit. Most two hundred hour programs cost between $3000 and $4000; however, it is important to consider additional costs over and above the tuition. For example the Bikram teacher training [www. bikramyoga.com] costs more than $6,500 for a nine-week immersion, and people who don't live in the Los Angeles area generally spend more than $3500 in hotel costs.

Location

If you don't live in a larger city, the chances are you will have to travel. Maybe you will spend six months living in New York, Los Angeles or San Francisco. Perhaps the thought of staying in the Berkshire Mountains at the Kripalu Ashram [ww.kripalu.org] sounds nice—or maybe you want to travel to someplace tropical to study. There are many options, but if you are going to travel it is important to factor travel costs, food, and lodging into your budget. Also, if you plan to travel outside your own country for the training, it is important to know what travel documents you need (e.g., passport and visa), as well as the vaccinations and shots recommended by your health care provider.

Continuing Education

Even if you have completed a teacher training program of 200 or 500 hours, it is essential that you continue your education. The practice of yoga is nothing if not vast, and the teacher who believes he or she is no longer a student is not much of a teacher at all.

Remember, you are always a student first. Teaching is nothing more than sharing what you have learned and integrating it into your own practice. Of course every one of us is different and we will all be drawn to focus on different aspects of yoga.

For example, Jane Austin [www.janeaustinyoga.com], a popular teacher in San Francisco, has incorporated her training as a midwife into her work with pregnant and new mothers by offering classes in pre and postnatal yoga. She even offers a hugely popular "Mom and Baby" class.

Kimberly Wilson [www.kimberlywilson.com], a well-known Washington, DC teacher, has focused much of her attention on empowering women. In her book, *The Hip Tranquil Chick,* she seeks to help women move their practice off the mat and into just about every aspect of life, including mindful shopping and conscious party planning.

While Kimberly and Jane have taken very different approaches to working with women, both have one important thing in common: They are both very dedicated to continuing their own studies. Neither of them would simply sit back and say, "Okay, I'm done studying now; I can move on to teaching." Aside from growing as yogis, this keeps their classes fresh, new, and exciting for their students, so people keep coming back.

Continuing education can come in many forms. You may choose to study consistently with one teacher, or you may want to shop around and take workshops from a variety of senior instructors. If you live in a major city, you may want to take workshops from a number of guest teachers who pass through town, or you may need to travel to study at a retreat center or ashram for a week or two every year.

The Yoga Alliance requires all registered yoga teachers to complete continuing education hours every year. You can learn more about their continuing education requirements at their website. www.yogaalliance.org

> *Beginners acquire new theories and techniques until their minds are cluttered with options. Advanced students forget their many options. They allow the theories and techniques that they have learned to recede into the background. Learn to un-clutter your mind. Learn to simplify your work. As you rely less and less on knowing what to do, your work will become more direct and more powerful. You will discover that the quality of your consciousness is more potent than any technique or theory or interpretation. Learn how fruitful the blocked group or individual suddenly becomes when you give up trying to do just the right thing.* —*John Heider,* THE TAO OF LEADERSHIP

Personal Reflections

◊ How much time am I willing to commit to a training?

◊ Am I willing to give up my weekends in order to become a yoga teacher?

◊ Am I willing to go away for two weeks or a month to become a yoga teacher?

◊ What style of yoga do I most want to teach?

◊ What training fits my schedule?

◊ How much can I afford to pay for this education?

◊ Where would I like to study?

◊ Do I have the necessary travel documents for leaving my country?

◊ Have I consulted my health care provider regarding the physical challenges of the training, as well as the medical concerns regarding travel to certain areas?

Part Two:
The Yogi Entrepreneur

The Buddha said to Ananda: "Truly, Ananda, it's not easy to teach the way of freedom to others. In teaching freedom to others, the best way is to first establish five things and then teach. What are the five? When you teach others, you must think:

I will teach in a gradual and sensitive way.

I will speak with the goal in mind.

I will speak with gentleness.

I will not speak in order to gain anything.

I will not speak with a view to harming anyone.

If you establish these five things, your teaching will be well received."

—Gotama the Buddha, *The Anguttara Nikaya*

CHAPTER 3:
FINDING A JOB

The first thing necessary for yoga is concentration of purpose. You have so many aims, so many purposes, that you are frittering away your little stock of energy in the attempt to accomplish them all. You are pursuing so many objects not because they are pleasant or profitable in themselves, but because you have not yet found the highest good of your life. —*Sri Ananda Acharya*

The Job Hunt

On any given night my classes range from forty to sixty students. I have written books on yoga, led retreats, and traveled throughout the United States and abroad to teach and lecture. By any measure, I have become successful as a yoga teacher.

However, this success did not come easily. It took a lot of hard work and has been a slow but steady uphill climb. In the beginning, I worked hard to find students and had to convince gyms that hiring me would be good for their membership quotas. I had to learn through trial and error that being a successful yoga teacher means really working.

The good news is that that the demand for yoga has grown and continues to grow, and this makes finding a job teaching much easier. The bad news is there are so many teacher training programs pumping out teachers that competition can be stiff.

In this chapter, I would like to look at three basic ways of earning a living as a new yoga teacher. In later chapters we will look at some additional ways to expand your teaching and your opportunities for earning money doing what you love, but for now let's keep it simple.

A Brief History of the Yoga Craze

When I first started teaching yoga in 1990, things were much different. Gyms were very reluctant to offer yoga classes, as they seemed too hokey and new age, and there were very few yoga studios. Also, the numbers of people interested in taking yoga was miniscule compared with today.

Thus, if you wanted to teach yoga, chances are you worked for yourself. Perhaps you hosted a weekly class in your living room, or maybe you rented out a small room at a local church, community center, or library. Whatever the case, you were expected to do everything, including marketing the class, collecting money, paying rent, insurance and other expenses, buying props and other supplies, signing students into class, and then of course, teaching.

At that time, you felt like the King of Siam if you had ten students on a regular basis, and if you were able to do that during two or three classes per week, you were a standout in the fledgling yoga community. Then, over the course of five or six years, something happened that changed the yoga community forever.

First, Jane Fonda, who had become synonymous with home workout videos, started promoting yoga over aerobics. Instantly, thousands of middle-aged women who had come to trust her on matters of physical fitness began to flock to yoga classes. A few years after that, pop icon Madonna, began to tout yoga's benefits, and with that a whole wave of other celebrities began talking about it. Suddenly a surge of younger women were rolling out their mats along side the middle-aged crowd. The final trigger in the massive wave of yoga came when popular sports teams began to incorporate yoga into their training regimen. All of a sudden a flood of men began to attend classes as well.

As all of this happened, the demand for yoga increased exponentially, and the venues for teaching also increased. Gyms were the first to recognize that offering yoga classes was a great way to attract new members. When I first started teaching at the Market Street Gym in San Francisco, [Market Street Gym was later purchased by Gold's Gym. www.goldsgym.com] the management was reluctant to give me a prime time slot for teaching. Being new to the area, I was grateful to have the opportunity to teach at 7:00 a.m. on Tuesdays. I wasn't sure if anyone would even show up, but the club members were so hungry for yoga that the class quickly filled, and the management then added a number of additional classes during prime time slots. The same gym, now under new management, is considering adding an additional room that will be dedicated solely to yoga, to meet the ever-growing demand for more classes.

As my students at the gym grew in number, it became apparent that teaching yoga full-time was something I wanted to do more. It was at this time that more yoga studios were beginning to pop up in large cities. Beryl Bender Berch's book, *Power Yoga*, was selling like hotcakes and many people were turning to yoga as their main source of exercise rather than an add-on to support other types of workouts.

This brings us to today and to the subject of this chapter—finding a job! As the profession of teaching yoga has evolved here in the West, it has grown like a large snowball picking up various facets along the way. Let's take a moment to look at each one.

Gyms and Fitness Centers

A great place to start working is at a local gym. Not only do they have a built-in audience for you to teach, but they also provide a regular source of income for new teachers who have not yet built a name in the yoga world. There are a few things to consider about gyms, however.

Unlike many yoga studios, gyms are all about fitness. If your thing is chanting, displaying a photo of your guru or giving a ten-minute talk on yoga philosophy at the start of your class, you may make some gym members uncomfortable, as well as the management.

While many gym yoga students grow into great yogis over time, the majority are coming to class for purely physical reasons in the beginning. Thus, lighting candles, dimming the lights, burning incense and chanting to Krishna, is usually a great way to get fired. Some gyms even have a policy against promoting the spiritual aspect of yoga.

That said, take heart in knowing that while your class may not have the spiritual overtones that a private or studio class would offer, it is a great way to introduce large numbers of people to yoga, and from a business perspective, it is a great way to build your following and market other workshops, events, and retreats that you may choose to offer once your student base has grown

Another great perk associated with working at a gym is that there is no financial risk to you. If you show up at a class and no one is there, you don't have rent to pay. In fact, most gyms pay a flat hourly rate for their teachers, so you will likely make guaranteed money whether you have any students or not. Once your classes grow and you have a large following, this may not be to your advantage, but in the beginning, it can provide a nice safety net.

Though every gym is different, most pay yoga teachers as independent contractors. When we talk about accounting, you will want to pay attention to this, because it will affect how you file your taxes.

While gyms tend to have lower standards for who they hire (when compared to yoga studios) most will want to see that you have at least two hundred hours of training, that you are a member of *The Yoga Alliance*, and that you have liability insurance.

Questions to Ponder

◊ How large is my student base? (The smaller your student base, the more likely you will benefit from working at a gym.)

◊ How much does the gym pay?

◊ How do they pay? (flat hourly rate, per student, etc.)

◊ Will the gym let me market myself? (hand out schedules, announce workshops, have a mailing list, etc.)

◊ Do I get a free gym membership while working there?

◊ What types of members does the gym attract? (body builders, women, gay men, seniors, etc.)

◊ Will the gym allow me to blend spiritual elements into my teaching?

The Yoga Studio

As a general rule, finding work at a yoga studio is more difficult than at a gym, because the managers of yoga studios, as well as their students, are more discerning about the teachers with whom they will work. Also, yoga studio managers like to know that you are bringing students with you.

If you are fresh out of teacher training and have no experience, this tells studio managers three things: First, you are untested, second, you don't have a following, and third, as a new teacher, you still have a lot of growing to do. Given the competitive nature of yoga studios—especially in cities where there seems to be a studio on every block, you will be hard pressed to find a studio willing to take a gamble on you.

But don't lose all hope. There are a number of things you can do to increase your chances of being hired, though it may take time and persistence. The following three tips will go a long way in putting you on the radar while at the same time giving you some much needed experience.

Sean Haleen [www.seanhaleen.com] was new to the very saturated market of San Francisco in 2010 and he wanted to work at Yoga Tree [www.yogatreesf.com]. Because Yoga Tree is the city's largest studio, teaching positions are very coveted. Many people have tried, unsuccessfully, to garner a teaching position at this renowned center.

But Sean had two things that many other teachers don't have—self-confidence and determination.

He had developed self-confidence by studying hard and committing himself to a near constant stream of continuing education after his initial training. He didn't simply finish a 200-hour program and call it quits.

His determination was rooted in the understanding that if he were going to get a job at such a well established yoga studio, he would need to stay on the radar. Tara, the owner of Yoga Tree, is one of the sweetest women in San Francisco, but because of her prominence in the yoga community, many teachers freeze up like star struck fools when they meet her.

If Sean was nervous around Tara, he never let it show. He befriended her, took her classes and she even had the occasion to see him at a number of trainings with their mutual teacher, John Friend.

Now there is nothing insincere about Sean. On the one hand he genuinely likes Tara and respects everything she has done to advance yoga in San Francisco, but on the other hand, he believes in himself and he is never afraid to remind Tara that he really wanted to work for Yoga Tree.

Within a year of Tara hiring him, he had become one of Yoga Tree's most sought-after teachers, and Tara often remarks on how happy she is to have him working for her. The difference between Sean and many other teachers is that Sean believed in himself and his actions clearly reflected that.

Studio owners like Tara want to hire people who will work hard and represent the center into which they have poured so much passion.

Ask yourself this: If you owned a studio, would you hire someone like Sean, or someone who comes across as either entitled, or insecure?

1. Work At a Gym

As I noted above, getting a regular teaching job at a gym is much easier, and while it gives you some guaranteed money, it also gives you much needed experience, as well as a great opportunity to build your mailing list.

2. Assist Senior Teachers

If there is a teacher you like and respect—a teacher whose style is similar to what you envision yourself teaching—approach them and ask if you can assist them with their classes. Or better yet, ask if they will mentor you. This puts you on the radar with not only their students, but also the studio management, and you will learn a great deal about their teaching methodology, assisting, and teaching techniques.

3. Substitute Teach

Find out what the requirements are for substitute teaching at the studios in your area, and get on their sub lists. Then take classes from teachers with whom you share a similar style and remind them regularly that you are available. Many teachers are busy, and spending hours looking for subs is never fun. Most teachers will call the people who are consistently available, so make sure to eagerly say yes whenever asked. If students compliment you after subbing a class, politely invite them to drop the management a note commenting on their experience.

CHAPTER 4:
GETTING PAID

*The real measure of your wealth is how much you'd be worth
if you lost all your money.* —*Author Unknown*

Every studio is different when it comes to compensation. Some will pay a
flat rate much like gyms. Others pay a per student rate, and still others do a
combination of the two by offering teachers a flat rate for teaching the class
and a smaller per student bonus.

Like gyms, most studios will pay you as an independent contractor rather
than an employee; however, this is starting to change as the IRS has been
cracking down on yoga studios that have full-time employees.

Self-Employment

If you are really independent and willing to do the leg work, there is no
reason you can't simply start your own classes by renting a space and
marketing your class. This, of course, takes a lot of work and commitment,
so be prepared! Consider your options and the amount of time and effort
you want to put into building a class (or a number of classes).

First, look at the costs involved. You will likely need to rent a space, and
if you are teaching from your home, you will need to be sure you carry
the proper insurance (more on that later). Since you will be paying money
out, it is important to make sure you will be earning enough to cover your
expenses, as well as to pay yourself for your time and efforts.

For example, let's assume you are going to teach an eight-week class at a
studio space you are renting, and you can reasonably expect ten students to
take the class. The spread below is an example of how things might work
out. Keep in mind that there are a number of variables (such as the cost of
renting the studio). Thus you will need to do your own spread sheet for an
accurate total amount.

EXPENSE	AMOUNT	NOTES
STUDIO RENTAL	$600	$75 PER WEEK X 8 WEEKS
MARKETING	$80	POSTCARDS, FLYERS, WEBSITE ETC.
INSURANCE	$20	
TOTAL	$700	
10 STUDENTS	$960	10 STUDENTS X $12 PER CLASS FOR 8 WEEKS
EARNINGS	$260	GROSS - EXPENSES

As you can see, there is a lot of work involved with no guarantee and some risk. If you rent the space and only three people show up, you will be losing money. On the other hand, if you can increase your attendance to fifteen people, your revenue goes up significantly. This is because your expenses are largely fixed. The hall rental, for example, will be the same regardless of how many people register.

Pros and Cons of Self Employment

Pros

◊ Control over what you teach

◊ Control over who you teach

◊ Potential to earn more

◊ Develop a deeper relationship with your students

Cons

◊ Financial Risk

◊ Much more administrative and marketing legwork

◊ Greater legal liability

◊ Potential to earn less

CHAPTER 5:
PROFESSIONAL ETHICS

Real integrity is doing the right thing, knowing that nobody's going to know whether you did it or not.—Oprah Winfrey

There is nothing more important to a yoga teacher than his or her reputation. In order to teach poses, breathing techniques, and meditation effectively, students need to trust their teacher. Yoga is, of course, much more than a glorified stretching class. It is a tool for healing and a system of radical personal transformation. In order for that process to occur, a relationship of utmost trust and respect needs to be cultivated between teacher and student.

Students need to know that the vulnerable places to which we guide them, the very places where profound healing and spiritual growth take place, will not be abused by us. Without trust they will not experience the comfort and safety to truly let go.

In addition to the individual relationship you form with your students, you also represent our profession. How you behave and the ethical standards you choose to follow or ignore, affect yoga teachers everywhere. Every time a yoga teacher acts unethically, the reputation of our entire profession is diminished.

The child abuse scandal in the Catholic Church is one such example of this principle. While the vast majority of Catholic priests are good men who only want to support their parishioners spiritually, some have acted out in very immoral and unethical ways. What was once viewed as a noble profession quickly became tainted by the inappropriate behavior of a few and the institutionalized cover up of these criminal and immoral acts that followed.

A friend of mine, Father Mike, who is a delightful man and a fantastic priest, is constantly met with skepticism from parents in his parish because of the stain left on the church by a relative few priests who were allowed to harm children by the hierarchy. While most priests are like Father Mike, they will, for years to come, have to bear the burden inflicted on their profession by this scandal. Worse still, many of the people they had hoped to guide spiritually will not feel comfortable seeking them out or placing trust in their hands.

As yoga teachers it is essential that we act from a place of honor. Sadly we are getting a reputation for being loose with our professional ethics, and it has affected the way we do business. Paul Keegan wrote an article for the website Business 2.0 entitled *Yogis Behaving Badly*, which is required reading for anyone going through the teacher training program I run at Yoga Tree in San Francisco.

In his article, he lists numerous well-known yoga teachers and gurus who have done very unsavory things. In the process, the five moral precepts (yamas), all yogis strive to live by, not to mention the professional ethics that all professionals are expected to observe, were disregarded. Unfortunately, this has resulted in the entire yoga profession losing credibility.

Like any professional, a yoga teacher is in a position of power. Just as a doctor, a lawyer, a psychotherapist, and an accountant needs to be trusted by their clients in order to be of any help, so too, yoga teachers need to be trustworthy.

All professionals are expected to follow a code of ethics that guides how they behave with their clients. The ethics may change marginally from profession to profession, but the basic principles are the same. In fact, not following strict ethical guidelines is the fastest way to be excommunicated from the professional groups that oversee each profession. Lawyers can get disbarred for disclosing confidential information about their clients, psychotherapists will quickly lose their license for inappropriate sexual contact with clients, and false or misleading advertising about cures will certainly cost a doctor his or her license.

As yoga teachers, we also need to follow certain guidelines. Let's discuss in some detail what those ethics are and how best to observe them as yoga professionals.

Sexual Conduct

Several years ago I led a retreat to India. After the closing circle, a young woman approached me and gave me a big hug. She had tears in her eyes and she said that she wanted to thank me. Retreats can be powerful and moving experiences for many people, so gratitude is not uncommon.

Her gratitude was not for the reasons I had expected, however. "I want to thank you for being gay," she said as her eyes filled with tears again.

Over the years I have heard a lot, but this statement knocked me back on my heels. It must have shown on my face because her tears quickly turned to laughter.

"Thanks," I said, " but I'm not sure I can take credit for that. It is certainly not something I planned. It just sort of happened that way."

Jennifer was a very attractive woman by conventional standards and I'm sure she receives a lot of attention from heterosexual men. The problem was that she was receiving too much inappropriate attention from male yoga teachers, and when she signed up for my retreat she feared that she would have to spend the whole retreat fending off my advances. Once she learned that I had no interest in her in that way, she was able to relax and go deep into her practice.

Another student, Kelly, overheard our conversation and chimed in. Kelly was attractive as well, but she was slightly overweight. "I have to agree with Jennifer. I'm so tired of going to yoga classes where the pretty girls get all the attention, and fat girls like me are invisible to the teacher. One of the reasons I come to your class, Darren, is that I know you are not there to hit on the pretty girls. I know that you are there to work with everyone."

I was honored that Jennifer and Kelly both felt safe and cared for in my class, but the conversation left me feeling very sad for my profession in general, and for male yoga teachers in particular. The truth is that my sexual orientation has nothing to do with the way I treat my students. In truth, most straight male yoga teachers don't hit on their female students, but it happens often enough that many women complain.

Yoga teachers of all stripes, gay and straight, male and female, have acted out in this way, and it is exceedingly damaging. Teaching yoga is one of the few professions left, in which we are allowed to touch our clients. Even when you go to the doctor or dentist, there is generally a latex glove between you and the doctor.

Thus, yoga is a powerful way for people to receive healthy, therapeutic and non-sexual touch in a safe environment. Far too many people in our culture are touch-deprived. We desperately need to experience nurturing, non-sexual touch and either consciously or unconsciously, we seek out yoga for that very reason.

If you taint the experience of yoga by sexualizing your class, you are doing a great disservice to your students, which could take years to undo. This is not to say that sex should be treated as a dirty or bad thing, but it has absolutely no place between you and your students.

> *Yet our freedom should not be used as a reckless license to do anything we please. In true freedom and happiness, we like whatever we do, but we do not always do whatever we like. —Swami Nirmalananda*

Five Things to Remember

1. Comments about a person's physique, either positive or negative, will set a tone of judgment in your class.

2. Showing added attention to students to whom you are attracted will make them uncomfortable and will alienate the other students as well.

3. Students know when you are copping a feel rather than providing them with a healthy and therapeutic adjustment. The intention behind the touch will always shine through, so keep your focus on the task at hand, rather than groping.

4. Flirting is never appropriate. Even if the student tries to flirt with you first, it is not acceptable for you to return the flirtation. It is not uncommon for students to develop a crush on their teacher. This is never an excuse for you to flirt with, or worse, sleep with that student—EVER!

5. If you are considering dating a student, STOP. Students, like children, are off limits. There are rare circumstances in which a genuine, loving, adult relationship may be appropriate, but this must be considered in the most careful way possible.

The Question of Love

When I give talks about yoga teacher ethics, I inevitably get questions about genuine love rather than a purely physical attraction. This of course makes for a very thorny issue. Before we delve into specific circumstances, I think we need to be very clear about the various types of attraction.

Physical Attraction

No doubt students will come into your class who will catch your eye because of their physical beauty and/or their sexual energy. The fact that someone is physically attractive is NEVER an excuse to flirt, ask them out, touch them in inappropriate ways, or engage in sexual activity. The fact that you are physically attracted to someone is not a license to be inappropriate.

Emotional Attraction

As yoga teachers we are naturally predisposed to helping people. Our students are often grateful for our help and the result can be an emotional bond. This emotional bond is akin to the bond a child may feel for an adult mentor, and as such is NEVER an excuse to engage in sexual activity.

According to psychiatrist Eric Berne, who developed the psychological theory of Transactional Analysis, we take on one of three roles in any relationship. The three roles are "the parent," "the adult," and "the child." For example, you may find yourself dating someone who is very parental at times or you may find that you tend to be the parent and they tend to be the child. You may have a very playful and child-child relationship with your best friend, in which you laugh and joke, and you may have an adult-adult relationship with another friend.

Most relationships are a mix of things. Sometimes you may play the role of the parent and your partner may play the role of the child, while at other times that role may be reversed. Sometimes you may interact as two adults or perhaps as two children. These changing roles are healthy and should be expected.

In almost all cases, the student-teacher relationship is one in which the teacher takes on an adult or parental role and the student takes on the role of a child; it is in this unconscious role playing that the student-teacher relationship is most therapeutic.

As each of us develop during the first few years of life, a pattern emerges between the infant and his or her primary caregiver. A need arises, such as hunger, or the need to have a diaper changed. We cry out for help, and our caregiver responds to that need. As the need is satisfied, a deep bond develops, and each time this pattern repeats itself that bond deepens.

In a perfect world, all of our needs are met adequately and in a timely manner. But none of us live in a perfect world and no parent or caregiver is perfect either. Thus, patterns emerge deep in the psyche that reflect the level to which our needs were met. In the case of severe abuse and neglect, the resulting patterns can be quite dysfunctional. Even in the best of situations, our caregivers make mistakes. Consequently, all of us bear the scars of unmet needs from early in life, and therapeutic relationships such as the one between a doctor and patient, a psychotherapist and client, or a yoga teacher and student, become a powerful tool for healing those unmet needs.

In order for the therapeutic relationship to be effective, we need to understand this very natural dynamic. The fact that a student may be sexually or romantically attracted to you is almost always a result of patterns that were developed early in life. While this is a natural process in which great healing can occur, there is also risk involved. When you are in the role of teacher, flirting with, dating, or becoming sexually involved with a student prevents the therapeutic relationship from forming. In fact, these inappropriate behaviors may very well deepen the psychological wounds from their formative years.

A number of years ago, when I was still practicing massage therapy, a woman came to me for bodywork on a weekly basis. Megan was a very attractive woman who had physically developed at an early age, and received a lot of unhealthy attention from the boys in her class. Not only that, her stepfather was also extremely inappropriate with her. As an adult, Megan worked as both an erotic dancer and an escort. In short, the only attention she was used to getting from men was the objectification of her body.

From our very first session, Megan experienced strong emotional release. Sometimes the tears would flow uncontrollably. Other times she would softy cry. It was clear that much of her trauma was being released by receiving healthy touch that was nonsexual. After about a month, Megan sheepishly asked me if she could make me dinner as a thank you for all I had done, and before I could even answer, she said, "and maybe a little something more than just dinner."

Naturally I declined and explained to her that while I was flattered, I had a rule about socializing with clients, and it would be unethical for me to get involved with her. She began to sob. When she finally calmed down, she thanked me for being a gentleman.

Things would have unfolded much differently had I taken Megan up on her offer. The therapeutic benefits she was getting from the bodywork would have stopped, and the progress we had made would have quickly been reversed. In addition, I would have proven to her, like so many men before me, that she was an object and nothing more.

Occasionally a student may come to your class and an adult-adult relationship will form. A genuinely loving romantic relationship may begin to develop. In these very rare cases, it is important that we proceed with the greatest of caution. If you truly believe that the feelings you are experiencing are real and adult-adult in nature, it is important to take the following steps:

1. Consider that your feelings may not be rooted in adult love, but rather in physical attraction or the need to 'save' or fix someone. When strong attachments form, the ego can be very convincing.

2. If, after deep soul searching, you are convinced that your feelings are rooted in an adult-adult attraction, it is time to talk to a neutral party— perhaps another yoga teacher who shares your values, or your supervisor at the studio or gym where you teach. This third party will have the benefit of seeing the situation absent of the oft-blinding effects of an attraction.

3. If, after you complete the two steps above, you decide that you would like to pursue a romantic relationship, it is time to talk to your student and tell him/her how you are feeling. He/she may return the feelings

or not share your attraction, but it is important that you make it clear that the nature of your relationship is changing, regardless of how he/she might feel about you, as he/she will need to find another teacher, for a time. It's inappropriate to continue teaching someone for whom you have romantic feelings.

Romantic and sexual attractions are very complicated. Certainly, if you look back over your life you will probably see that many of your most foolish mistakes were made when you were sexually aroused or experiencing deep romantic feelings. We are all human and this is natural, but as natural as this experience may be, we as yoga professionals, need to act responsibly. Failure to do so will result in tarnishing your reputation and the reputation of our profession. Most importantly, the wellbeing of your students is compromised.

> *Never forget that you are in a position of power as a yoga teacher. Students come to you trusting that you will not abuse that power. Your primary job as a yoga teacher is to build a safe and trusting relationship with your students. It is essential for the welfare of your students, your own personal reputation, and the reputation of our profession that you NOT violate that trust.*

Confidentiality

My friend and fellow yoga teacher, John, once had a female student, Melissa, tell him that she was pregnant. Although she was early in her pregnancy, she wanted to make sure she did not do anything that would harm the baby. John advised her about the various precautions and went on to teach the class.

Later that day, he was talking with a friend and told him about Melissa's pregnancy. What John didn't realize is that his friend had recently started dating Melissa, and did not know she was pregnant. Because their relationship was new, Melissa was still in the process of sorting things out before she told him.

Naturally, this created a very awkward situation, and while John was not speaking out of malice, he was breaking a very basic rule of professional ethics—confidentiality.

Students will frequently share all sorts of information with their teachers. Some of it is based on medical conditions, while other details may be rooted in the emotional and psychological issues that bubble to the surface as a result of the practice. Any detail shared with you by a student, however small, must be kept in the strictest of confidence. These details are not to be shared with anyone, including your friends or your romantic partner, without permission from the student.

Points to Remember

1. Never share details about a student without their permission.

2. Ask about injuries and medical conditions in a way that allows for privacy.

3. Even seemingly good news (pregnancy, a new job, engagements, etc.) are details you do not have the right to share without permission.

4. If you need advice about how to address students' unique needs, change the details enough to protect their confidentiality.

5. When working with students in the context of a public class, check in with them quietly so that you are not announcing their issue to others.

Exceptions to the Rule

There are only two times when it is acceptable to break confidentiality. The first is if the student is going to hurt him or herself. The second is if the student is planning to hurt another person. In these two cases, and these two cases only, it is important to share this information with the appropriate authorities.

> *Right speech is speech that furthers the practice of the speaker and contributes to the well-being of others and the world. Right speech is therefore intentional speech that rejects mindless chatter, gossip, slander, and lies. When we are honest with ourselves, self-reflection often reveals that much of our speech is harmful at worst and unnecessary at best.*
> *—Judith Hanson Lasater & Ike K. Lasater,*
> What We Say Matters: Practicing Nonviolent Communication

Non-Discrimination

Our world is filled with prejudice, and some of the greatest evils in human history have been rooted in discrimination. Yoga should always be a hate-free zone. To treat people of any race, ethnicity, national origin, sexual orientation, gender, gender identity, or religion, with anything but the deepest respect, is both unethical and not in keeping with the principles of yoga.

It's one thing to offer a specialty class for a particular group, such as a women's group or a group for a particular sub-culture, but it is an entirely different thing to prevent a certain group of people from attending your class.

Of course, most discrimination is not overt. I don't know of any white supremacists teaching yoga. But there are subtle and not so subtle ways that teachers can make individuals or groups of people feel uncomfortable.

Here in San Francisco, for example, you will occasionally hear a disparaging comment about political or religious conservatives. Certainly it is no secret that San Francisco is a very liberal city, and the teachers and students here tend to reflect a more progressive point of view. But making unwelcoming comments about other groups, not only makes those minority groups feel uncomfortable, it establishes an atmosphere of judgment. In truth, everyone can benefit from yoga, and to subtly not invite a particular group, sets a very bad tone.

A few years ago, one of my students, Vivian, brought her mother to my restorative class. I didn't think much of it, as a lot of avid yoga students want to bring their parents to yoga, and the more athletic styles would not be suitable. After class, her mother thanked me and gave me a big hug. She seemed like a very sweet woman, and I was happy to have her there.

About a week later, Vivian came back to my class and asked to speak with me afterward. "Thank you so much for being so kind to my mother," she began. "I was raised in a very conservative Christian home, and my mother has been worried about me ever since I started yoga. She was afraid I was getting involved in a cult or something. Anyway, I brought her to your class because I knew she would feel safe and that your style would not threaten her beliefs. She told me after the class that she took the quiet time during deep relaxation to pray and that she had never felt closer to Jesus. She was so excited to find a class when she returned home to Arkansas."

Can you imagine what this woman's reaction would have been if I had made a disparaging comment about her faith? It most likely would have turned her off from yoga forever and would potentially have created a rift between her and Vivian. By simply providing a warm and welcoming environment, two lives were changed for the better.

Accurate Advertising

There is a saying in the medical profession, "Don't be the hammer that only sees the nail." What this means is that because a hammer is a tool used to pound nails, it can easily see everything through that tunnel vision

As yoga teachers, it can be easy to think that yoga is good for every situation, and to be sure, it is helpful for a lot. But to assume that yoga is a miracle cure for every ill, is dangerous and unethical.

Sometimes I find myself at the local cafe or health food store, reading over the yoga flyers that are posted there, and I'm often shocked by the exaggerated claims that some teachers make. In some cases, the claims are blatantly false and even dangerous. In other cases, the claims are exaggerations.

The truth is that yoga is a profound and life-changing practice. It is helpful, directly or indirectly, for many issues, and there is absolutely no reason to exaggerate or make unrealistic promises.

There's a studio in San Francisco that used to post photos of famous people in their window. They didn't actually come out and say, "These celebrities practice our studio," but that was certainly the implication. Of course some people fell for this ploy, but most people discovered this was just a gimmick and quickly found other studios at which to practice at. False or misleading advertising may seem to pay off in the beginning, but eventually people will catch on and no longer take you or your teaching seriously.

When you advertise, keep the following points in mind:

1 Never make false or misleading claims.

2. Never make negative comments about other teachers or other healing modalities.

3. Always be clear about the cost of the class or workshop you are offering.

Money

For some reason, money seems to challenge yoga teachers more than any other issue. Culturally speaking, we think nothing of paying huge sums of money to entertainers, professional athletes, and the CEOs of large companies, who pay little regard to improving the world and see the bottom line as the only measure of worthiness. Yet, some hold the view that a healer, spiritual teacher, or minister, should work for free or charge close to nothing for their services.

I have a policy never to turn people away because of money. If a student can't afford my class or workshop, I find a work/trade situation. If they can't do that, I ask them to "pay it forward" by giving something to someone else when they can.

Several years ago, I was teaching a class for people who are HIV+. The cost of the class was set below what most yoga classes cost. As I was hanging a flyer in a local cafe for the class, a man approached me and was visibly angry. "I think it is outrageous that you charge HIV+ people for your classes!" Before I could reply, he stormed off in a huff.

Had he given me the chance I would have invited him to take the class for free if he couldn't afford it. But since he didn't even bother to let me respond, I was not very inspired to chase after him. It's unfortunate that his views about money reflect the way many people feel, including many yoga teachers.

Much healing needs to be done around money if we are to be mindful business people. Learning to face our issues about money head on will insure that we will make an honorable living, while at the same time insuring we are not making money the reason we teach. The following principles should be considered carefully.

Capitalism versus Commercialism

Many people confuse the terms capitalism and commercialism. Capitalism operates on the law of supply and demand. If there is a need (demand) and you can answer that need (supply) you will be very successful in your business. People need health, spiritual nourishment, and a safe place to deal with the stresses of life. If you can answer that need with a quality yoga class, workshop, or retreat, people will flock to you.

Commercialism is all about manufacturing a need where one doesn't exist. For example: "If you want men to find you attractive, you need to wear that makeup," or "If you want women to find you attractive, you need to drink this brand of beer," and so on. It is important that we not fall into this trap as yoga teachers. People genuinely need what yoga offers. This is not to say that yoga is the only way to fill those needs, but it is certainly a very effective answer to those basic human requirements.

Therefore, we don't need to manufacture reasons for people to take yoga. By simply providing a safe space, quality instruction, and an invitation to wholeness, people will come of their own accord. Better still, they will keep coming. On the other hand, if you resort to commercialism, people will soon tire of your work and will go on to look for the next best thing.

> *Funny thing about guilt— There's nothing so bad that you can't add a little guilt to it and make it worse. But there's nothing so good that you can't add a little guilt to it and make it better. Guilt distracts us from a greater Truth— That we have an inherent ability to heal. We seem intent on living through even the worst heartbreak.*
> —C. Jay Cox (From the Movie , LATTER DAYS)

Scarcity and Abundance

The Yogic texts teach us that this universe is an abundant one. We don't always get what we ask for, but we always get what we need. Living under the umbrella of abundance ensures that you will always have enough. Living under the tyranny of the ego ensures that you will never have enough.

The Devil card in the tarot deck often depicts tortured souls trapped in hell. It's interesting to note that they are free to leave anytime if they simply let go of the treasure chest that they are all clinging to. Scarcity is never about how much money you have in your pocket. There are people who have millions of dollars and spend their lives in fear of losing it.

Likewise, there are people who have almost nothing, yet live in peace because they trust that if they do the right thing—if they live their dharma—their needs will be met. As yoga teachers, we need to do our work from a place of abundance rather than scarcity. Not only is it the ethical thing to do, but also it makes good business sense. If you are continually worried about money, your students will sense that and will be repelled. However, if you approach your teaching from a place of abundance, students will sense that and will be drawn to your classes in droves.

A Fair Price for a Quality Product

Finding a fair price for what you sell is essential. Many people are surprised to find that my retreats are so affordable, especially when you compare my rates to the rates of other teachers. What is most interesting is that my retreats always sell out, and in the long run, I tend to make more than many of my cohorts.

It's easy to get caught up in the false belief that the more you charge, the more you will earn. Frequently, charging a little less will make your work available to more people and the result is often a much larger revenue stream. I'm not suggesting that you give your services away—just that you consider how much you are charging. For example, if you are offering a weekend retreat, you could charge $300 or $500. At $300, many more people will be able to afford the retreat. Thus, at $500 you may only have ten participants, pulling in $5000, whereas at $300 you will likely double the number of people who attend, pulling in $6000. You win because you pulled in more money. They win because they can afford to spend the weekend healing through the practice of yoga.

It's not Yours to Sell

In the past few years there has been a rather sad attempt by some in the yoga community to copyright various aspects of the practice. Yoga poses and Sanskrit words have been around for thousands of years and have been handed down from teacher to student through various lineages. To think that any one individual or group has a monopoly on yoga is both arrogant and unethical.

As you venture out into the world to share yoga with people, remember that it is merely on loan to you. True, you will be giving the practice your own personal spin and style, which will appeal to some and not to others, but the practice is much bigger than you.

It is for this reason that all teachers need to be ever mindful that what we are doing for livelihood must be a gift that is freely given. While we need to take care of ourselves and meet our basic needs, yoga should always be available to everyone who wants it, regardless of their ability to pay.

With this in mind, consider how you will make your teaching more accessible. Perhaps through a work/trade program, scholarships, or even pro-bono work. While teaching yoga can be a wonderful way to support yourself, it's not yours to sell. To deny people yoga because of money is unethical and ultimately cheapens the practice.

Paying the Rent Enables You to Reach More People

Money is a difficult issue for many of us—not just in terms of accounting and taxes, but because we need to find a healthy and ethical way of paying for our basic living expenses, while at the same time ensuring that money is never a deterrent for anyone who seriously wants to practice yoga.

Making an honest, above board living teaching yoga enables you to reach more people and to extend yoga's reach. Your ability to pay the rent, put food on your table, and provide for your family, creates more space in which to share your practice with the world.

This is not to say that you will be rich. Indeed, the choice to teach yoga often requires a more austere lifestyle, but that doesn't mean you should ignore your own needs. In many ways we need to think of yoga the way we are instructed to think of the other passengers on an airplane. Just as it is important to make sure you put your own oxygen mask on before helping others, we need to make sure our basic needs are being met before we can do an adequate job of supporting others in their practice.

Time

Start your class on time to show your respect for the practice; end your class on time to show your respect for your students. —Judith Hanson Lasater

Have you ever arrived on time for a doctor's appointment only to have the doctor keep you waiting? How did that make you feel? One of the most unprofessional things a teacher can do is ignore a person's time. Just as the doctor who is late for your appointment is viewed in a negative light, so too are yoga teachers who fail to understand that most students have very full lives.

Time is a valuable resource, but unlike most other resources, you cannot get it back once it is gone. If I were to steal the twenty dollars in your wallet, that would be a bummer, but you could always go out and earn more money. If I steal or waste your time, you can never recover that loss.

Maybe a student had to rush from work to get to your class, or maybe they are paying a babysitter by the hour. Maybe they worked really hard to carve out an hour and a half to take a yoga class. Whatever the case, dishonoring a student by starting your class late or failing to end your class on time is both unprofessional and unethical.

There is one studio in San Francisco that boasts some really talented teachers. Yet several years ago I stopped going to that studio because classes never started or ended on time. Teachers would continually go well beyond the scheduled end time for their class and would usually leave the practice room a sweaty mess for the following class. Worse still, it was not just one teacher who did this—the studio management allowed for a culture in which this lack of attention to time was viewed as an acceptable norm.

I spoke to the owner about this once, and his response was, "Live and let live. . ." It was then that I decided that I would never attend a class at that studio again. And while I kept this opinion to myself, I often heard others complain about this blatant disregard for time.

I have a policy to start and end my classes on time, and students really appreciate this. They can plan their day around my class because they know exactly when the class will begin and when it will end. This is, in my view, very much in keeping with yogic principles as well as professional ethics. While it may be tempting to think this is a far less important tenet of yoga teacher ethics, paying attention to time is one of the best ways you can create a safe space in which people can really relax into the practice, because they don't need to worry about when the class will begin and end.

Remember:

◊ Your class should always start and end on time.

◊ Deep relaxation is part of your class. . . Not an encore.

◊ Putting away props is part of the practice. If you use props, budget time for clean up.

◊ Dry mopping the floor is part of your class—not the class that follows yours.

◊ If another class is starting shortly after yours, invite your students to take conversations out of the practice room. Respecting the time of other teachers is also part of professional ethics.

Whatever enchants, also guides and protects. Passionately obsessed by anything we love—sailboats, airplanes, ideas—an avalanche of magic flattens the way ahead, levels rules, reasons, dissents... bears us with it over chasms, fears, doubts.—Richard Bach "THE BRIDGE ACROSS FOREVER"

Chapter 6:
Accounting, Taxes, Insurance and Bookkeeping

*It's income tax time again, Americans: time to gather up
those receipts, get out those tax forms, sharpen up that
pencil, and stab yourself in the aorta.—Dave Barry*

Yoga teachers may be known for a lot of things, but finance is not one of them. Many of us are actually repelled by the notion of balancing a checkbook, let alone bookkeeping and taxes. As I write this chapter, I'm feeling much of your pain. As much as I love my accountant, I dread going to see her every year because numbers and accounting make my head hurt.

That said, I have learned a lot over the years and have found that a few basic things have made the whole experience much easier. In fact, once I learned a few things about accounting, I started saving thousands of dollars each year on my taxes. So as much as you might be tempted to skip to the next chapter, I think you will find it worth your while to consider the following tips.

IMPORTANT REMINDER While I hope this chapter is helpful, it is not substitute for an accountant. Laws vary from state to state and from country to country and change all the time. Please use this chapter as a loose guide only and consult a qualified professional regarding your unique needs.

Sole Proprietorship & Independent Contracting

For the purposes of taxes there are numerous ways to earn money and thus file with the federal government. Let's take a look at two of the most common ways in which yoga teachers earn money.

Employee

Some yoga teachers are employees of the studio or gym in which they work. What this means is that out of each paycheck, your employer will withhold some money to cover your various taxes. These taxes include estimated income taxes, Social Security, disability and Medicare, as well as state taxes.

There are benefits to being an employee, and a few drawbacks too. First, if you don't like accounting, your employer will do much of that for you. They will deduct the money before you ever see it, and send it to the federal and state government. Hopefully, at the end of the year, they will have taken out enough money that you don't owe any additional taxes.

In addition, your employer will pay half of your FICA and Medicare (about 7.65% at the time of this writing). What this means is that unlike the self-employed person, who pays the full amount as a self-employment tax, you will only have to pay half and your employer will match that. Basically, it is like getting a small raise. Of course, this number can change and may be higher in other countries or depending on where you reside.

In the United States, your employer is also required to pay Worker's Compensation insurance, so that if you get injured <u>on the job</u>, you may receive money each month. Naturally the laws change, so be sure to check with your state in order to more fully understand your rights.

The drawback to being an employee is that you cannot itemize business expenses. Itemizing is a great perk, as we shall see shortly.

Sole Proprietorship

It is no secret that most employers would love to get out of paying half your Social Security tax, Worker's Compensation, and other fees associated with employing people. Therefore many yoga studios and gyms will hire you as an independent contractor.

The drawbacks here are clear. If you don't like saving your receipts and doing bookkeeping, then being a sole proprietor is not to your advantage. However, if you are willing to keep track of your business expenses and take responsibility for your own business, then you can come out way ahead.

As an employee, your employer may take care of many of your accounting headaches and pay half of your Social Security tax, but your hands are largely tied with regard to business write-offs. As a sole proprietor, you are able to write off just about everything, which can reduce your tax burden considerably.

The Middle Path

Many yoga teachers hold more than one job. Either they work nine to five and then teach yoga a few nights per week, or they work at multiple studios or gyms. This can make organizing your accounting complicated, as each place of employment may be compensating you in a different way. It is for this reason that having a good accountant you trust is essential.

Filing your personal taxes as an employee is usually fairly straightforward, so I'm going to focus the remainder of this chapter on filing as a sole proprietor. If you are an employee, there are many accountants qualified to help you. There are also several computer software programs, which can assist you in filing and declaring personal deductions.

> *Worried about an IRS audit? Avoid what's called a red flag. That's something the IRS always looks for. For example, say you have some money left in your bank account after paying taxes. That's a red flag.*
> *—Jay Leno*

Quarterly Taxes

If you are self-employed, every three months, you are expected to send the Federal government a check for your estimated taxes. This may seem a bit unfair, as employees don't have to do that. But in truth, they do. Their employer is taking money out of each check and sending it in for them.

If you are not an employee, you need to do that for yourself. If you overpay, you get a check back at the end of the year after you file your taxes. If you underpay, you will not only owe that money, but you will also most likely get hit with a fine for not pre-paying enough.

Unless the figures are way off, the IRS will usually let it slide if you are paying based on the previous year's taxes. If, however, you start making a lot more, you will need to account for the increased income or the IRS can fine you. In the United States (at the time of this writing) quarterly taxes are due on the 15th of April, June, September and January. In addition, most states require self-employed people to pay quarterly taxes. Your accountant can advise you on the laws in your area.

The 30% Rule

There is no way to know how much you will owe in taxes each year until you sit down and focus on the books. If you are good at bookkeeping, you will be able to estimate that as you go along. As you file from year to year, you will have a much better idea of how much to pay each quarter, but until then, you should plan to put at least 30% of your total income aside to make sure that at the end of each quarter, you are not caught short. Again, this a general rule, so please be sure to discuss this with a certified public accountant.

> *The hardest thing in the world to understand is the income tax.*
> *—Albert Einstein*

Accountants: Angels from God

To make money, you should never be afraid to invest, and the best investment you can make is in a good accountant.

Years ago I did my taxes myself with the help of a computer program. This got the job done, and it was rather inexpensive to buy the software. The problem was that my tax bill each year was an extremely high percentage of my income. Then a fellow yoga teacher told me about his accountant and suggested I give her a try.

When I first spoke with her on the phone, she explained to me that her fee for filing my tax return would be between $300 and $500, and that would depend on how many hours my particular situation would take.

I really didn't think I could afford her, but I was tired of getting soaked every year by the IRS. So I did my best to lock my frugal nature away temporarily.

That first year, I showed up with a large envelope filled with receipts, which took the two of us hours to go through. This pushed my bill closer to the $500 mark. That said, she saved me nearly $5000 in taxes that first year alone.

The following year I returned, a bit more organized, and not only was her bill less, she was able to save me even more. This trend has continued year after year. Not once has she failed to save me thousands of dollars, and she's worth every penny I pay her.

Tips for Working with an Accountant

1. Always find a Certified Public Accountant. (Your best friend may be cheaper, but is not properly trained in the many details of tax law.)

2. Get organized. If you come with a shoebox full of receipts, your accountant is going to charge you more and likely miss some valuable deductions and business expenses.

3. Choose the right accountant. Like most professionals, accountants specialize—some in corporate accounting, others in small businesses, and others in sole proprietorship. Depending on your needs, as well as the needs of your spouse if you have one, you will want to consider the types of clients with which your accountant is most skilled.

Accounting and Bookkeeping Software

Perhaps the best thing you can do to support your accountant is to get accounting software for your Macintosh or PC. This will reduce the amount you pay the accountant in tax preparation fees. The most popular software is Quicken, but there are others as well. All of them do roughly the same thing. You simply set up accounts, such as checking, savings, credit card, and cash, and then you log all the activity within each account.

This may sound daunting, but it is actually quite easy. Start by making a list of all the accounts you have with various banks. Most banks will allow you to download your transactions to make data entry simpler.

Once the transactions are downloaded into the various accounts, you can assign each transaction a category and sub-category. When it comes time to do your taxes, you simply press a button and print out a report to hand to your accountant. It's also a good idea to give them a digital file as well.

Getting set up is the hardest part. If you are feeling overwhelmed, you can always hire a bookkeeper to do the initial set up and show you how to work the software.

Personal Finance versus Bookkeeping Software

Quicken, Microsoft Money, iBank, and other personal finance programs will likely be all you need—at least in the beginning. However, should your business grow, you may want to consider bookkeeping software such as QuickBooks or MYOB AccountEdge.

The main difference between the two, is that bookkeeping software allows you to keep track of things like payroll, retail inventory, and client accounts. Again, it is highly unlikely that you will need such advanced software initially, but your accountant and/or bookkeeper can advise you on this.

Tip: Before you buy accounting software of any kind, be sure to contact your bank and make sure the software you want to buy is compatible with your accounts. While you are on the phone with them, find out how to download transactions and how much they charge for that service. Usually it is between five and ten dollars per month, but every bank is different.

Business Expenses

It would be impossible for me to list all the business expenses you can and cannot write off. My personal policy is to keep track of every penny I spend, and then let my accountant decide what is an expense and what isn't.

It's also important to note that not all expenses are dollar for dollar. For example, a business meal is only a percentage of the bill, and your auto expenses are only for miles between job sites—not between home and work. Your accountant will guide you through these complex formulas.

That said, here is a sample list of what you may be able to write off. Your unique circumstances will certainly add additional write offs. Likewise, not all of these may apply to you.

◊ Computer

◊ Mobile Phone

◊ iPod

◊ Yoga Music

◊ Yoga Books

◊ Yoga Props

◊ Continuing Education

◊ Professional Insurance

◊ Automotive Expenses

◊ Travel Expenses

◊ Teaching Supplies

◊ Stationery

◊ Postage

◊ Accountant & Bank Fees

◊ Yoga Alliance Membership

◊ Internet and Website

◊ Business & Travel Meals

◊ Charitable Donations

On my income tax 1040 it says 'Check this box if you are blind.' I wanted to put a check mark about three inches away.—Tom Lehrer

Ask the Professional

To better help you understand the process of accounting and taxes, I asked Sean Tiret, a certified public accountant who works with a number of yoga teachers, if he would address a few of the most common questions new yoga teachers ask [smtiret@gmail.com].

Q: **With so many different types of accountants specializing in different types of accounting, which qualities do you want your accountant to have?**

A: A yoga teacher will want an accountant who specializes in individual and small business accounting and taxation. Apart from general bookkeeping and tax return preparation, other services to consider when choosing an accountant would be financial statement preparation and analysis, small business consulting, retirement plan consulting, and financial planning.

Q: **What accounting software do you recommend?**

A: I would recommend either Quicken or QuickBooks. Quicken is designed as a personal finance software, and is generally more user friendly for someone with little or no accounting knowledge. QuickBooks is more comprehensive from an accounting standpoint and is geared more toward small businesses than individuals. Whichever software program you choose to use, or even if you don't use one, make sure you save your receipts, bank statements, and other supporting documentation for your business income and expenses for a **minimum** of three years from the date you file your tax return. The IRS has a statue of limitations of three years for Federal Tax returns. Depending on your resident state, you may need to save them even longer. (California's general statute of limitations for assessment of tax is currently four years from the date the return is filed.)

Q: **What are some of your favorite deductions for yoga teachers?**

A: Some deductions to consider if you are working as an independent contractor (self-employed) are as follows:

Health insurance – if you are self-employed and pay for health insurance, you can take a deduction on your tax return for the annual cost of the insurance (although, this cannot reduce your net income below zero).

Home office – this is a somewhat prickly subject with the IRS; however, if you are self-employed and don't have a studio or other outside office you use, you may be able to take deductions related to a home office. This would include the portion of your rent, utilities, maid service, internet, phone, etc., allocable to your home office using a square footage ratio. The IRS has fairly stringent guidelines on what constitutes a home office, so make sure you are familiar with these before taking the deduction.

Cell phone – if you use your cell phone for business, the business percentage of your bill is a deductible expense.

Continuing education – classes and workshops attended to enhance your knowledge of the profession are a deductible business expense.

Auto – this can be calculated two ways; either using actual expenses for gas, oil, repairs, etc., multiplied by a business use percentage (business miles divided by total miles driven for the year), or by multiplying your business miles by the IRS's standard mileage rate applicable for the taxable year. All tolls and parking expenses incurred for business travel are 100% deductible. Annual depreciation can also be taken on your vehicle if it is used as a business asset.

One thing to note is that most deductions are not black and white. There are many expenses that may be deductible to one taxpayer, but not necessarily for another. If you are in doubt as to what constitutes a valid deduction, you should consider asking/hiring an expert.

Q: **What is the difference between an accountant and a bookkeeper and how important is it to have both?**

A: Bookkeeping is a specific type of accounting service. A bookkeeper organizes your financial activity into a useful format (usually in the form of financial statements). An accountant is a broader, all-encompassing term that would describe someone who provides one or more services, such as financial statement preparation and analysis, audit services, bookkeeping, tax preparation, tax consulting, retirement plan consulting, and estate planning, to name a few. At the minimum, a yoga teacher is going to want someone who provides tax return preparation. Bookkeeping is a function a yoga teacher can do on his or her own using basic accounting software and gathering some basic accounting knowledge. As a business grows in activity and complexity, it might make sense to hire a bookkeeper so that more time is spent concentrating on the yoga side of the practice, rather than getting overwhelmed with the financial side. Additionally, as the practice grows, it would be a good idea to incorporate tax planning, retirement, and business consulting.

Q: **What is the difference between an employee and an independent contractor, and are there advantages and/or disadvantages to both?**

A: The Internal Revenue Service (IRS) classifies someone as an employee when the employer controls what work will be done, when it will be done, and how it will be done. An individual is classified as an independent contractor when the person for whom the services are performed is only controlling the end result of the work, and not how or when the work will be done. Whether or not you are paid as an employee or an independent contractor will usually come down to how the individual or company hiring you interprets the nature of your employment. If you are on the hiring side, it would be best to discuss the decision to treat individuals as employees or independent contractors with an accountant familiar in this area of practice.

When you are classified as an employee, your employer will withhold from your paycheck federal and state income taxes, federal social security tax, Medicare tax, etc. Additionally, your employer will pay certain payroll taxes for employing you. When you are classified as an independent contractor, no taxes are withheld from your paycheck. Instead, you are required to make federal and state quarterly estimated tax payments. As an independent contractor, a self-employment tax will be assessed on your tax return in addition to income taxes.

If you are paid as an employee, you cannot directly deduct business expenses against your employment income. The idea is that since you are an employee of a business, your employer should be paying or reimbursing you for all necessary business expenses. The only way to deduct expenses as an employee is to treat them as unreimbursed employee business expenses. Unreimbursed employee business expenses are only deductible if you itemize deductions by filing Schedule A with your tax return, and they are only deductible to the extent they exceed 2% of your adjusted gross income.

If you are paid as an independent contractor, you can directly deduct business expenses against your business income. Other items that are deductible if you are self-employed are health insurance costs and one-half of the self-employment tax assessed on your tax return.

Q: Can you explain some of the basic tax forms a yoga teacher will need?

A: If you are being hired as an employee, you will be completing Form W-4, which tells your employer how much federal and state income tax to withhold from your paychecks, based on certain factors such as the number of dependents you claim on your tax return, marital status, and whether or not you itemize deductions. Shortly after the end of each year you are employed, you will receive a Form W-2, which contains your annual earnings and tax withholding information for use in preparing your federal and state tax returns.

As an independent contractor, you will complete Form W-9 at the beginning of your contract, which gives the individual or business using your services information necessary for them to issue a Form 1099-MISC. After the end of each year for which you were working as an independent contractor, you will receive a copy of the 1099-MISC, which will report the total amount paid to you for the year. (**Note:** current law only requires 1099-MISCs to be issued if an independent contractor was paid $600 or more during a taxable year.)

Q: Does the IRS tend to audit yoga teachers and what should a person do if he or she is audited?

A: In general, a person's chance of being audited is very low. In past years the IRS has audited less than 2% of individual tax returns. With that in mind, self-employed individuals are a high-risk audit area, so if an individual is being paid as an independent contractor, then they would be at a slightly higher risk of being audited.

If you are one of the lucky few selected by the IRS for audit, don't panic. If you prepared the return yourself, go back through each line on your return and make sure you have documentation supporting the numbers. Make sure everything is organized and easy to review prior to the date of the audit. If there are some areas of confusion, or you're not quite sure you understand the tax law, you might consider hiring a tax accountant to help you with the audit. If you hired an outside tax preparer to prepare your return, contact them and let them know you were selected for audit. Most tax preparers have their own process to prepare for the audit. In my firm, we have the auditor come to our office for the audit so it is not intimidating or inconvenient for the client.

Q: If a person has multiple sources of income such as a 9-to-5 job and teaches yoga part-time, what accounting advice do you have for them?

A: This comes down to the nature of the person's employment with respect to both jobs. If the individual is classified as an employee for both their 9-to-5 job and yoga teaching job, then there is not much complexity from an accounting and tax standpoint with respect to both these jobs. One thing to watch out for when you have multiple jobs is that, depending on your total income for the year, you do not have too much Social Security tax withheld for the year, since there is an income cap on the amount of Social Security tax owed for the year. Some state taxes, such as California's disability tax, also have an income cap and should be considered as well.

If the individual is classified as an independent contractor for one or both jobs, then they should consider the various points discussed throughout the rest of this interview. It would also be important to keep separate records for each business.

Chapter 7:
Leading Workshops and Retreats

Our deepest fear is not that we are inadequate. Our deepest fear is that we are powerful beyond measure. It is our light, not our darkness that most frightens us. We ask ourselves, Who am I to be brilliant, gorgeous, talented, fabulous? Actually, who are you not to be? You are a child of God. Your playing small does not serve the world. There is nothing enlightened about shrinking so that other people won't feel insecure around you. We are all meant to shine, as children do. We were born to make manifest the glory of God that is within us. It is not just in some of us; it is in everyone. And as we let our own light shine, we unconsciously give other people permission to do the same. As we are liberated from our own fear, our presence automatically liberates others.
—*Marianne Williamson*, A Return To Love: Reflections on the Principles of A Course in Miracles

In the beginning, you will want to focus on building regular classes at local gyms and yoga studios. Eventually, you will build a following of students who will want more of what you have to offer. Your unique style and personality will attract a number of people who will want more than you can provide them in a standard class. Thus, workshops and retreats are wonderful ways to support your students and earn more money.

Workshops

A workshop can focus on any aspect of yoga, such as alignment principles, yoga philosophy, anatomy, a special needs issue, or even teaching skills. Whatever the topic, a workshop is a great way to take students to a deeper place than a regular class allows. It's also a way to specialize your teaching and generate more income.

Les Leventhal [www.yogawithles.com], a popular teacher in San Francisco, offers regular workshops on yoga and the Twelve Steps. In doing this, he is helping many people throughout the city to explore the natural connection between their Twelve-Step recovery work and the practice of yoga. In addition, he has made a name for himself in the recovery community as a teacher who can support its specific needs. This not only brings many people to his workshops, but also makes him much more attractive as a teacher to a specific audience.

Facilitating a workshop is different than teaching your standard yoga class, however. One of the big mistakes many new teachers make is the assumption that a yoga workshop is little more than a longer yoga practice. This always results in students feeling disappointed. A workshop is a time to break down concepts and techniques that are difficult to teach in a regular class; so when planning a workshop, a few pedagogic principles should be observed.

There are many forms of pedagogy, which is the art and science of planning a curriculum that will take students from a lesser level of understanding to a higher level of understanding. In an academic setting, pedagogy is most often focused on intellectual development, but the same principles can be applied to the physical and emotional levels of our being.

Pedagogy is not something that can be taught in a few pages here in this book, as it is something that educational professionals spend years studying and cultivating. But a few key principles are worth considering as you plan a workshop. Asking yourself the following questions as you plan your workshop will help you present one that will set yours apart from the plethora of other yoga teachers out there offering similar things.

Who is my audience?

To know your audience is perhaps the most important thing you can do. If your audience is all new students and you try to teach them headstands, you will lose (and perhaps injure) them. If, on the other hand, your audience is more advanced, they will quickly get bored if you focus on topics they already know.

Knowing your audience will help you in preparing your promotional material, developing your talking points, coming up with suitable exercises, and speaking in a language that they can easily understand. Many people skip right over this very important question and wind up losing their students immediately.

For example I sometimes teach anatomy classes for yoga teachers. My anatomy class is much different for them than it would be if I were lecturing to medical students. My focus is different—the examples I use come from yoga practice, and the exercises we do to solidify that the information I have given is tailored to yoga teachers. The workshop would be quite different if I were speaking to a different audience, even though the topic is the same.

What do I want to teach my audience?

This may seem like a silly question, but it is one that goes unanswered by a great many teachers. Either they try to cram every point they have ever learned about yoga into that one workshop, or they jump around from point to point with no order, reason, or logic.

In any workshop, you should have five or six key points that you want to make and no more. For example, if I were teaching a yoga workshop on the spine, I might want to focus on the six movements of the spine. First, I would discuss lateral flexion to the left and right and then discuss some of the benefits and precautions of that type of movement. I would do the same for forward bending, back-bending, and twisting.

Following this, I would have them practice yoga, and I would focus the sequence and my comments on the specific movements discussed. This would give them a real and tangible experience of the concepts we discussed.

In doing this, the six movements of the spine would become concrete and useful for them. Rather than focusing on every aspect of the spine and its movements, I have simplified it to make it useable, real, and comprehensible.

What key points do I want students to take away from the workshop?

In a three-hour workshop, it's unlikely that any more than three or four points will be truly integrated into the student's life or practice. By clarifying in your own mind what those points are, and then reaffirming those key points in a variety of ways, using examples and exercises, students will be able to take away certain nuggets of information. This is, of course, far more effective then spewing out a number of random facts and hoping that something sticks.

What examples and anecdotes can I offer that will help to solidify those points and make them meaningful?

The first time I took algebra in high school, my teacher was dry and boring. The class was painful and even the math geeks in the class were fighting back the onset of the REM cycle. Because math is not my strong suit, I had the joy of taking the class again.

Luckily, when I took the class the following year, I had a teacher who made it useful. She didn't simply give us problems to solve but made those problems relevant to our young teenage lives. She used humor and anecdotes that we could relate to. The semester flew by, and I actually learned more about algebra than I ever thought possible.

More importantly, I learned something about teaching. People learn much more easily when they can relate to the information being presented. When I wrote my second book, *Yoga and the Path of the Urban Mystic*, I had one primary goal in mind. I wanted to make the often-complex principles of yoga philosophy meaningful for yogis in the modern world. Certainly there are many books that are more extensive than mine with regard to their content, but if the average reader falls asleep reading the first page, then little has been gained. Thus, giving meaningful examples will increase the retention of whatever you are teaching.

What activities and exercises can I offer to make the key points real and meaningful?

Yoga is nothing if not practical. In fact, it's often referred to as a 'science' for that reason. If you are teaching a workshop, be sure to include poses, breathing techniques, and meditations that reaffirm the key points you are trying to convey.

I could lecture all day about the benefits of inversion poses, but it's not until I actually put someone upside down that they begin to feel those benefits. By feeling something in the body, it becomes a solid and real experience that the student can draw on in the future.

What handouts and other resources can I provide so students can review the information in the days and weeks that follow the workshop? What homework can I give students at the conclusion of the workshop to help them refine and practice their newfound skills?

Over the years I have taken many workshops and the ones that stick out in my memory the most are the ones that stick with me. They don't just pump information into my head, but rather they stimulate me to think, and I'm inspired to practice in a new way.

As yoga teachers our goal should always be to have the workshop experience extend beyond the end of the workshop. One way to do this is to give the students handouts to review at home, or to provide them with resources so they can investigate the topic more on their own.

Another thing you can do is offer homework. If you just taught a workshop in breathing, ask people to really notice their breath as they practice the following week; or if you just taught a meditation workshop, invite people to practice meditation every morning for a week, so they can feel the long-term effects of meditation when practiced over the course of time.

Remember, if you have done your job, you not only gave the students valuable information, but you also inspired them to deepen their practice in some way. In effect, you have helped them to raise their sails. Offering them some concrete yet attainable homework exercises will fill those sails with wind!

Getting Paid for Workshops

Like standard yoga classes, there are a number of ways to get paid for yoga workshops.

Commission Based Teaching

For most teachers this is the most efficient way to operate. Generally you will hold your workshop at a gym or yoga studio, and then take a percentage of the money collected. This ensures that the studio or gym providing the space will help with the marketing, and in many cases they will handle registration and the collection of money.

For example, imagine you were teaching a three-hour workshop on back-bending. For this workshop you are charging $30 in advance, and $40 at the door. You have ten students pre-register, and three students simply show up. The total income would be $420 ($30 x 10 = $300 plus $40 x 3 = $120).

Most studios offer a 50/50 split for newer teachers and a 60/40 split for more advanced teachers. Teachers with more seniority may even demand a larger cut. For the sake of this example, however, we will assume you are collecting 50% of the gross giving you $210 for your workshop.

Do It Yourself Teaching

If you decide to go it alone, you may make more money, but you could also take a loss. Let's use the example above and look at it from the "do it yourself" point of view. In order to pull this off, you will need to find a facility in which to hold your workshop. At $75 per hour (and it might be a lot more than that) you would need to earn $225 just to pay your rent. In addition, you would need to do all your own marketing and registration, which can be costly in terms of time, as well as money.

The bad news is that if you have the same ten students show up and you gross $420 for the workshop, you will make less money than if you had done a 50/50 split with a local studio. The good news is that if you have fifteen people attend, you will earn quite a bit more than you might at the studio. The catch is that you have to feel very confident about your ability to attract enough students to make it work.

Five Tips for a Successful Workshop
◊ Encourage or require preregistration.
◊ Don't over plan.
◊ Always give students time to share.
◊ Offer 'homework' and handouts to help students apply what they learned.
◊ Know your subject!

Tip for Registration

Whether you are leading a workshop or a retreat, you will need to register students. In many cases, the yoga studio hosting the event will handle registration, but if you need to do this yourself, there are two great online resources that can make the process effortless.

Online Registration

If your registration needs are fairly basic, www.HeartBeat.com has a very simple and user-friendly interface for handling the registration of workshops and other events. Another good option is www.ConstantContact.com, which can also manage your email list. If you need something more advanced, www.MindBodyOnline.com may be a better choice. While the MindBody software was originally designed to run yoga studios, they also have packages for individual teachers that are reasonably priced.

Leading Retreats

> *"Come to the edge," he said.*
> *They said, "We are afraid."*
> *Come to the edge," he said*
> *They came; he pushed them— They flew.*
> *—Guillaume Apollinaire*

According to yogic texts, our lives are largely governed by the ego, or in Sanskrit, ahamkara. The basic idea is that part of our mind incorrectly identifies with and attaches to false beliefs about who and what we are. In reality, we are powerful, eternal souls—sparks of the divine. But for most, the experience of that true nature is very elusive.

Rather than experience ourselves as infinitely powerful, we settle for the belief in littleness, and thus hold fast to the notion that we are weak and frail—that happiness and joy are temporary at best and dependent on external circumstances. Furthermore, the human ego knows, albeit unconsciously, that if we were to get quiet for any length of time, it would be revealed as a charlatan.

Thus, the goal of a yogi is simply to quiet the mind; it is in doing this that our true nature is revealed. At the start of a yoga practice, we experience this in small glimpses by simply attending yoga classes, but as time marches on we realize that we are doing the equivalent of a reverse Bunny Hop. For every step we take forward with the practice of yoga, we take two steps back as soon as we leave the yoga mat and return to the chaos that defines our daily lives.

This is where a yoga retreat can be a powerful and transformational tool. When we step out of our lives—when we remove many of the external distractions—we have the opportunity to go much deeper into the practice. Consequently, bringing a group of your students to a retreat center, a foreign country, or even out into nature, can be of great value to them. Doing this, however, requires particular care on your part, as your students will no doubt uncover much more on a retreat than they do in a standard yoga class.

In many ways, planning a retreat is much like planning a workshop, in that the experience should conform to the basic principles of pedagogy we discussed above. However, there are additional details that need to be considered.

IMPORTANT NOTE: When leading a retreat, remember that your job is much bigger than simply leading a couple of yoga classes. You are taking on a role as tour guide into the depths of the human heart and mind. Make sure you are prepared for people to release emotions, face difficult issues, and let go of long held patterns.

Facilitating this experience requires compassion, attentiveness, and being personally grounded. Before leading a retreat, it is essential that you remain strong in your own practice, mindful of the process that each student will likely go through, and never forget that your presence at the retreat is to hold a space for others, rather than to go on your own vacation.

To which population do I want to offer this retreat?

Not all yoga students are the same. Some have money, others not so much. Some will be drawn to a more plush retreat, while others will appreciate camping. Maybe you want to lead a men's retreat or a retreat for Christians who practice yoga. Perhaps you want to offer a retreat for couples, or maybe you want to market to the gay community. Knowing your audience will help you answer many of the questions that follow. Since each group will have unique needs, it's important that you consider this before you rush off and rent a retreat center.

Where will the retreat be held?

This seemingly simple question is perhaps the most important one. Unfortunately, many new teachers don't give it much thought. Choosing the right venue for the type of retreat you are going to lead is essential. If, for example your audience is wealthy housewives, they will likely want a spa-like setting that offers massage and has a hot tub. If, on the other hand, your group consists largely of college students on a limited budget, you will want to choose a venue with more affordable accommodations, such as camping and/or dorm rooms.

Another important consideration is the yoga room. If you plan to teach a prop intensive restorative class, you will want to make sure the center has props or you will need to make plans to bring your own. If you like to teach with music, what is the sound system like? Also, how many people can fit into the yoga room? Is there a way to adjust the temperature within the room according to the type of yoga you will teach?

What lodging will be available?

As a general rule, retreats that offer a wider variety of accommodations are easier to fill. For example, I often lead retreats at the Vajrapani Center [www.vajrapani.org] in the Santa Cruz mountains of California. The center is run by Tibetan Buddhists and offers everything from camping to private cabins.

The benefit of this is that it allows people on a budget to choose more modest accommodations, while people who prefer a bit more privacy and comfort, can choose a private room. This will make the retreat more inviting to a wider range of people, so filling the retreat is that much easier.

Who will provide the food?

I have led countless retreats and I have learned one very important thing—the way to a yogi's heart is through the stomach! If the food is good, I can botch up everything else and people will still be happy, but if the food is bad, it doesn't matter how flawless my teaching is, people will leave feeling miserable.

Sometimes the retreat center you rent will provide the food; other times you will need to hire your own cook. What is important is that the cooks know how to cater to your needs. If you are leading a vegetarian retreat, then the cooks should know a thing or two about cooking without meat. If you are focusing on a raw diet, the cooks should know how to plan a satisfying raw menu.

In addition, some of your participants may have unique dietary needs. If students are allergic to wheat or nuts, you need to know that, and you need to make sure the cooks you hire can accommodate them.

How will the various activities and workshops work together to complement each other and achieve the goals of the retreat?

A retreat is always greater than the sum of its parts. When I plan a retreat, everything is intentional. The opening circle and the closing circle are like bookends, and everything in between needs to be filled with the proper balance of yoga classes, workshops, and free time for personal reflection. Every detail is planned to take students deeper and deeper into whatever aspect of the yoga practice we are focusing on. Each class, workshop, and activity—the quotes I read, the chants we offer, and even the free time—are all strategically planned to bring students deeper and deeper.

A few years ago, I was leading a retreat in Costa Rica at a well-known yoga center called Pura Vida [www.rrresorts.com]. The focus of the retreat was to integrate philosophy with the physical practice of yoga. As a result, everything we did was designed to tie together various yoga principles with the physical practice.

Finally, it is generally not free for you to attend your own retreat. The base rates illustrated above likely apply to you as well. Most retreat centers will not give you free room and board, though there are some wonderful exceptions. For example, Aaron Star, the founder of Blue Osa Retreat Center in Costa Rica, will often offer free or reduced rates for teachers who bring groups to his facility. [www.blueosa.com]

That same week, a popular yoga teacher from Los Angeles, Vinnie Marino [www.vinniemarinoyoga.com], was also leading a retreat at Pura Vida. His group was focused on deepening physical poses. Thus, all of the work he was doing with his students was designed to take them deeper and deeper, and to explore advanced poses that are harder to practice in a standard class.

The two retreats, no doubt, looked very different. But they did share one thing in common. Both Vinnie and I had planned the retreats with very specific goals in mind, while the students were unaware of all the planning and thought that went into creating a complete experience. All the details were in place so that they could simply relax into everything and let the magic happen.

How will we develop a sense of community and a safe space?

At the closing circle of one of my retreats, a long time student, Philip shared something quite profound. He began his sharing by saying, "When I first arrived, I didn't like anyone here. I couldn't imagine what any of you had to offer me, and none of you seemed like people who held any interest for me."

There was a long, awkward silence before Philip continued. "But after spending four days with you all, I can't imagine not having known you. I feel closer to many in this group than I do to people I have known for years. I can't help but wonder how many people I overlook each day— on the bus, at work, and even in my own family—who are every bit as beautiful as each of you."

Philip had tapped into something very powerful on that retreat, and it is something that is very difficult to cultivate in a yoga class. There are few things more personal and more bonding than spiritual practice. Like sharing a meal or making love, shared prayer and meditation in any form is deeply bonding.

John Friend, the founder of Anusara Yoga [www.anusara.com], has recognized this and made the yogic concept of the 'Kula' or spiritual community a central tenet of that style of yoga. John has a deep appreciation for the ability of yoga to heal us on every level, and that includes the sociological level. Likewise, within the safety of a supportive Kula, the depths of the human heart and mind are much more easily reached.

On a retreat, there is a great opportunity for students to connect in ways that are not as easily accessible in a typical yoga class. The more you can do to encourage that group bonding, the deeper your students will be able to go.

> *If you can open to every person, emotion and situation without closing down, you will go as far as you can on the spiritual path, and will understand every spiritual teaching ever given.—Pema Chodron*

Tips for Building Community

◊ Allow time for people to share their experiences with the group or with others.

◊ Learn everyone's name and encourage everyone else to as well. Fun name games are a great way to accomplish this.

◊ Allow participants to help out. If people have simple jobs to do, they will feel more connected to the group.

◊ Facilitate trust building exercises, such as partner yoga poses. This invites people to trust the group in other, less tangible ways.

◊ Require confidentiality. If people know that what is shared in the group stays in the group, they will feel far more comfortable opening up.

How many participants are needed to break even? What is the maximum number of participants?

When we teach a yoga class and no one shows up, that can feel like a waste of time. It is not desirable, but it doesn't break the bank when it happens. When you lead a retreat, however, there is a considerable financial risk.

Most retreat centers will require a minimum number of participants, which means if they require ten people and you only register five, then you are paying for five people who are not attending. The same is usually true for cooks if you hire them. So before you do anything else, you should sit down with pencil and paper and figure out what your financial commitments are, how much you are going to charge for the retreat, and how many paying students you need to attend in order to break even.

Also, be sure to consider the capacity of the retreat. If the retreat center can only hold ten people and you need nine to just break even, then you are certainly not coming out ahead even if you completely sell out.

What is the refund policy?

Inevitably plans change and emergencies happen. People will sometimes register for your retreat and then need to cancel. Unlike a no-show for a regular yoga class, many cancellations will result in a loss of money for you. If you have paid for their room and board, or have turned others away as a result of holding a spot for them, this can get quite expensive. It is for this reason that I have a clearly stated "no refund policy." If there is a genuine emergency, I do my best to give full or partial refunds, but I never guarantee this.

Your decisions about cancellations and refunds will be a personal choice. However, whatever your policy is, be sure you state it clearly so that people will consider that when they register and before deciding to cancel.

What work, aside from teaching, needs to be done to make the retreat happen?

Many yoga teachers can teach on autopilot. We do it so much and so often, that we don't have to think much about it. Many of us teach at studios and gyms that even handle registration for our classes.

A retreat brings with it a number of responsibilities above and beyond teaching. In many ways you act as a travel agent, a cruise director, and a hotel manager. Students will need to plan their travel, which means packing their bags, getting driving directions and in some cases booking flights. They will need to be guided between classes, assisted with free-time activities, and locating their sleeping arrangements.

You will no doubt need to support participants when they are unhappy with a meal or their sleeping quarters, and you will have to be present for them should emotions arise as a result of intensive yoga practice. In short, you will be wearing many hats, and the more you can prepare yourself for this, the more smoothly the retreat will unfold.

Calculating the Costs

There are two main things you want to consider when calculating the cost of a retreat. What are the expenses per student and what is your time worth? Let's take each one separately.

Cost Per Student

Marketing, food, and lodging represent a significant cost. All of these need to be factored into the overall price to the participant. The following chart offers a sample of what you might expect to pay per student, based on their lodging requests.

LODGING	NIGHTLY RATE	NO. OF NIGHTS	LODGING SUBTOTAL	FOOD	MARKETING	TOTAL
CAMPING	$50	3	$150	$60	$15	$225
DORM	$75	3	$225	$60	$15	$300
BASIC ROOM (DOUBLE OCCUPANCY)	$100	3	$300	$60	$15	$375
DELUXE ROOM (DOUBLE OCCUPANCY)	$150	3	$450	$60	$15	$525
BASIC ROOM (SINGLE OCCUPANCY)	$150	3	$450	$60	$15	$525
DELUXE ROOM (SINGLE OCCUPANCY)	$200	3	$600	$60	$15	$675

Bear in mind that the above numbers do not include paying yourself. They are simply the costs associated with taking each person on a three night retreat. Also keep in mind that there may be additional expenses that are unique to your particular retreat.

Paying Yourself

Remember, a retreat is much more work than simply showing up to teach a yoga class. There is a huge amount of time that goes into writing promotional material, registering participants, writing and sending out confirmation letters, and arranging carpools. And all that is before the retreat even begins!

Once at the retreat you need to remember that you are always working. Students will want to talk with you during meals and will have questions about the issues that arise from the intensity of the practice. People will having lodging questions and will have forgotten to pack essentials, often expecting you to provide them. You may also be away from your regular classes or other job, so there will actually be a loss of income associated with just taking the time to lead the retreat.

Finally, it is not free for you to attend your own retreat. The base rates illustrated above apply to you as well. No retreat center will give you free room and board.

The Confirmation Letter

Crafting a detailed confirmation letter is essential. The more details you can include, the more a person can relax into the experience. Here are five things that every confirmation letter should contain.

◊ Packing List - What will they need to bring for clothing, toiletries, yoga props, and other supplies?

◊ Travel Instructions - Driving directions, carpooling information, which airport they should use, and what time to arrive.

◊ Emergency Contact - How can loved ones reach them in case of an emergency?

◊ Basic Scheduling - When and where will the retreat begin? What time will it end on the last day? What types of activities can they expect?

◊ Resources- Suggested reading, useful websites, and where to buy supplies.

Ask yourself the following questions:

◊ How much would I earn by staying home?

◊ What are my travel, food, and lodging expenses while on the retreat?

◊ How many hours will I need to invest over and above the actual retreat?

◊ What is my time worth?

◊ How many people can I reasonably expect to attend?

Once you have answered the above questions you can decide what your fee will be per student. There are two basic models. The first is based on a larger turnout and the second is based on a smaller turnout. The rule of thumb is this—the more people you have attend, the less you can charge and still make money.

If you have eight people attend, your expenses are going to be divided among eight people. If, however, you have twenty-five people attend, those same expenses are divided among a much larger number of people. Thus, you need to decide how many people you want to take, keeping in mind that a smaller group will feel much more intimate, while a larger group will have more energy.

If you want a larger group, it is wise to charge a bit less for the retreat. If, however, you want to have a smaller more intimate group, you will need to charge more. Finding that sweet spot at which people can afford to attend, while at the same time paying yourself a fair and living wage, can be tricky, and this is even more true during difficult economic times.

Now, using the numbers above, let's look at how you might price your retreat based on a few different scenarios.

Scenario One- 8 Students

LODGING	PER STUDENT	TEACHER FEE	TOTAL
CAMPING	$225	$200	$425
DORM	$300	$200	$500
BASIC ROOM (DOUBLE OCCUPANCY)	$375	$200	$575
DELUXE ROOM (DOUBLE OCCUPANCY)	$525	$200	$725
BASIC ROOM (SINGLE OCCUPANCY)	$525	$200	$725
DELUXE ROOM (SINGLE OCCUPANCY)	$675	$200	$875

TOTAL INCOME BASED ON EIGHT PAYING STUDENTS = $1600

Scenario Two- 15 Students

LODGING	PER STUDENT	TEACHER FEE	TOTAL
CAMPING	$225	$150	$375
DORM	$300	$150	$450
BASIC ROOM (DOUBLE OCCUPANCY)	$375	$150	$525
DELUXE ROOM (DOUBLE OCCUPANCY)	$525	$150	$525
BASIC ROOM (SINGLE OCCUPANCY)	$525	$150	$675
DELUXE ROOM (SINGLE OCCUPANCY)	$675	$150	$825

TOTAL INCOME BASED ON FIFTEEN PAYING STUDENTS $2250

Scenario Three- 20 Students

LODGING	PER STUDENT	TEACHER FEE	TOTAL
CAMPING	$225	$125	$350
DORM	$300	$125	$425
BASIC ROOM (DOUBLE OCCUPANCY)	$375	$125	$500
DELUXE ROOM (DOUBLE OCCUPANCY)	$525	$125	$650
BASIC ROOM (SINGLE OCCUPANCY)	$525	$125	$650
DELUXE ROOM (SINGLE OCCUPANCY)	$675	$125	$800

TOTAL INCOME BASED ON TWENTY PAYING STUDENTS $2500

All this is very important to consider because as you can see, charging less for a retreat, doesn't necessarily mean you are earning less. In fact, if you have more students, you will likely make more, and charging less will often make the retreat more accessible to a wider range of people. Of course, all the above numbers are hypothetical. Every retreat is going to be different, so you will need to sit down and calculate the amount you are going to charge for the retreat based on the costs per student, the number of people you can reasonably expect to attend, and the amount you need to earn to have your efforts match with the appropriate income. It's always better to estimate low and then hope attendance is high.

Tip: There is a point at which very few people will be able to afford your retreat. You may think your time is worth more, but the market may disagree. I have found that charging a little less and having a full retreat is often more satisfying and more financially sound. The best part is that your students can more easily afford to join you.

Housework is a breeze. Cooking is a pleasant diversion. Putting up a retaining wall is a lark. But teaching is like climbing a mountain.
—Fawn M. Brodie

CHAPTER 8:
PRIVATE SESSIONS

Yoga is like music, mathematics, art, or any other great tradition: you get from it what you put into it. If better health & a smaller waistline are all you want from Yoga, the class across the town will do just fine. And if you want to plumb the depths of Consciousness, understand the purpose of the universe, mitigate all material pain, attain spiritual bliss through self-realization, and have a personal rendezvous with God, you can get all that from Yoga too. But to cross that great ocean, prepare for a longer and more arduous voyage, perhaps decades in length. Arm yourself with good maps and plenty of supplies. And please: don't try to redesign the ship. It was wrought by a much better hand than ours.
—David B. Hughes

Working with groups can be very rewarding, but it also has limits. Some people need more individual attention, and this is where a private session can be very helpful. By working one-on-one, you can address the unique physical, emotional, and psychological needs of a given student in ways that are simply not appropriate, or not possible in the context of a larger group.

Rich was a regular student of mine for about six months before I saw him for a private session. He had started my restorative class at the suggestion of his psychotherapist, who had noticed that many of Rich's emotions were stored in his body. This made it very difficult for him to address those issues in their counseling sessions.

For six months, Rich would come to class, allow his body to open in the practice, and then go to his therapy session where he would have volumes to discuss with his therapist. In time, however, Rich felt the need to understand how and why the gentle yoga poses and breathing techniques were having such dramatic effects. He also wanted to deepen his home practice so he could accelerate his healing process.

Because his needs were both unique and private, he scheduled a private session with me to iron out some of the details. During our sessions we talked about some of the emotions that were coming up for him and why certain poses tended to affect him in certain ways. We also looked at poses he could do at home that would supplement his regular class practice, and I recommended some books for him that would cast a yogic light on his recovery process.

The work I did with Rich could never have been accomplished in a group setting, because his needs were both deeply personal and highly individualized.

There are a number of reasons why a student may need or want private yoga instruction, and all of them are valid. The question to ask yourself is, "Am I the best teacher for the job?" In order to answer that question, let's look at some of the reasons a person might seek out private yoga sessions. It's important to know why your client wants a private session so you can be sure you have the desire and the knowledge to give the experience he or she is seeking. Remember, it is always better to refer clients out if you don't have the skill-set or desire to help them.

Injuries and Medical Conditions

Many injuries and medical issues can be addressed by having a brief discussion with the student before class. You can quickly advise how to best modify the practice to reduce the risks of making the condition worse. You can also advise some yogic techniques to support them in their healing.

There are, however, some conditions that require much more time and attention. Several years ago, a good friend, Sean Cannon, discovered he had bone cancer in his leg. Chemotherapy and radiation proved unsuccessful in stopping the cancer, and in an attempt to prevent metastasis, his leg was amputated.

Once Sean somewhat recovered from the surgery and was fitted with a prosthetic leg, he wanted to begin a yoga practice. He was understandably worried about showing up to a class, so we met for a private session and explored his unique body issues. We came up with modifications on all the major poses that he could safely execute with his new leg, and we also worked on meditation and breathing techniques that would help him work through the trauma of having cancer and losing a limb.

Sean flourished in his yoga and soon started taking group classes. Unfortunately, the cancer did metastasize and Sean passed away in the summer of 2007. In spite of his shortened life, Sean was able realize many of his dreams, and his yoga practice was one small part of his ability to continue to live life to the fullest.

There are many people like Sean in this world who can benefit profoundly from yoga, but have specific injuries or medical conditions that make a group class inappropriate. Working with these individuals privately can be profoundly rewarding.

To Refine and Deepen One's Practice

A second group of people may want assistance in deepening their yoga practice. Perhaps they want to work on alignment, or want to better understand various breathing techniques. Maybe they want to learn the proper use of props, or they need help developing a home practice. Whatever the need, these basically healthy people simply want guidance on how to deepen their practice.

Shortly after I finished my training in massage therapy, I arranged to do a trade with my yoga teacher, Karen Lorienzo-Pratt. Although my body was young and healthy, I was surprised to see how quickly my postures improved by having her look at me in such detail. The subtle adjustments she made as I flowed through various poses dramatically increased my body awareness, and many of her tips and suggestions are still very much a part of my practice today.

Dislike Group Settings

Many people love the social aspects of yoga. They actively seek out classes that are chock full of people. There are, however, others who don't enjoy groups and find it very difficult to focus and relax when they practice in a group setting.

Still others are basically comfortable with groups, but in the beginning feel very awkward not knowing the basic postures. Once they are instructed in the basics, they will quickly move on to group classes. In the short term, however, they may benefit from one-on-one instruction.

Discuss Issues

It is no secret that yoga can bring up a lot of issues. In fact, many people have the experience of crying in yoga classes. While quite common and very normal, students want to know what is happening to them and why. Most people don't feel comfortable discussing these things in front of a room full of people. Thus, meeting with a yoga teacher privately can provide a space where they can share their concerns and get their questions answered.

It is important to note, however, that as yoga teachers, we are not psychotherapists, and we should not be attempting therapy. It is one thing to help a student understand the psychological and emotional release that yoga can evoke, but it is quite another to take on a role that you are not trained to undertake. When indicated, it is essential to refer students to the appropriate professional for proper diagnosis and therapy.

Developing a Yogic Lifestyle

Yoga is much more than the work we do on the yoga mat. When students are really serious about their yoga, they need to examine their entire lifestyle and make more balanced choices. A few years ago, I met with a woman who was struggling with her weight. While her asana practice was certainly helping her, she needed some guidance on how best to structure the rest of her life in general and her diet in particular.

On our first meeting we discussed her goals and mapped out a plan for her, which included quitting smoking and drinking coffee. This was followed several weeks later by modifying her diet and developing a home yoga practice. In fact, during one of our sessions we emptied her cupboards of all the junk food she had and donated it to the local homeless shelter. Then I took her to the local health food store where we stocked up on whole grains, organic vegetables, and other essentials.

Over the course of our time working together she began to lose weight, her skin conditions improved, and most importantly, she began to sport a contagious smile that brought regular praise from her friends, family, and co-workers.

Schedule Conflicts

Our modern lives can get quite busy. From time to time you may come across someone who really wants to study with you, but your regular class schedule will not fit his or hers. In these cases it can be helpful for you to work with them privately.

Fame and Fortune

For some people, money is no object, and for whatever reason they will simply be willing to pay for your private attention. My good friend Ryan Brewer [www.ryanbreweryoga.com] is a yoga teacher and personal trainer in Los Angeles. He has a large private practice in which he works with many movie stars and celebrities. Aside from having an abundance of money to spend, they also appreciate the privacy that working privately with Ryan affords.

For well-known people, attending public classes can often be less than relaxing, with people staring at them throughout the practice. Ryan honors their privacy and provides a space where they can practice away from the glare of the public spotlight; therefore, they appreciate the professionalism that he offers by keeping their work together confidential.

Charging for Your Time & Travel

Your time is worth something. Be sure you charge a fair price for your time, and that includes travel. Every minute you are teaching a private client or on your way to and from the session is a minute that you are unable to teach another class, enjoy some down time, or even do your own home practice.

In my experience, undercharging for private yoga sessions is a great way to be sure no one calls you. For the most part, people who can afford private sessions live under the belief that if they pay more for a service it is worth more. If someone is truly unable to pay, you can always charge less, but be sure to value your time, and never sell yourself short.

One cannot manage too many affairs: like pumpkins in the water, one pops up while you try to hold down the other.—Chinese Proverb

CHAPTER 9:
THE WANDERING YOGI

A few years ago I received an email from the general manager of CorePower Yoga [www.corepoweryoga.com], a rapidly growing chain of studios around the United States. CorePower Yoga used my book, *Yoga and the Path of the Urban Mystic*, as a required text in their teacher training program. They were wondering if I would be willing to visit each of their studios to teach workshops for their staff, their teachers in training, and their more advanced students.

That was the beginning of a very rewarding relationship with yoga communities around the country, with whom I would have never had the privilege of connecting, had I stayed in San Francisco exclusively. As my relationship with the CorePower Yoga chain of studios has grown, I've had the honor of connecting with their students around the country. Now I feel at home in Denver, Portland, or any of their other communities.

As my writing and my teaching became known beyond the San Francisco area, the connections I've made with studios around the world has grown, and I receive more requests to teach at studios outside of my hometown than I can handle. In the beginning I made a number of mistakes, because there were so many details that I failed to consider when traveling and teaching.

I can't help you avoid all pitfalls in one short chapter, but my hope is to offer a few things for your consideration, so you can avoid as much pain and hardship as possible. There is nothing more disappointing than flying across the country to have only three people show up for your workshop. In order to avoid this unfortunate scenario, consider the following:

Stand Out in the Crowd

What makes you unique as a teacher? Until you answer this question, you really have no business traveling and teaching. If your personal brand of teaching doesn't offer something unique to the offerings that already exist in the area where you're going, there is little or no incentive for the local yogis to take your workshop.

Identifying what you are offering and why you are a special and rare commodity, is something not easily done by new teachers. Most new teachers are still trying to find their voice. Their teaching largely consists of parroting what they have heard others say. But as a teacher grows and develops, he or she will become known for certain things.

For example, I'm known for my user-friendly approach to yoga philosophy, and I'm known for my work with cancer and HIV. Both of these qualities are not common traits among teachers in general. Therefore, when I travel, people take notice, because the workshops I'm offering are different enough that people want to work with me.

If I were to simply teach a vinyasa yoga class, I would be doing little more than competing with the other teachers at that studio. Studio managers know this, and most will not even consider bringing you in unless you have something unique to share at their center.

Local versus National Branding

When you consider teaching outside your local yoga community, you need to change your entire marketing strategy. Most people in New York City don't know much about the teachers in Los Angeles, even though they are quite popular on their home turf.

In fact, there are many fabulous yoga teachers all over the world who are basically unknown beyond their home town. Likewise, there are many well-known international yoga teachers who have built their followings on little more than hype and good marketing.

While it may seem unfair that some people with no talent become superstars, and many with talent are rarely recognized, it's a fact of life. The truly great traveling yogis need a little of both. To be really successful as a wondering yogi, you need to have both talent and some national, or even international, branding.

In addition to whatever talents I may have as a teacher, I have also worked hard to build a name for myself in broader circles. I have done this by hosting a popular blog, writing books, providing resources on my website, and podcasting talks and interviews that have international appeal.

Of course, these are not the only ways to brand yourself. Rodney Yee [www.yeeyoga.com] is famous for his high quality yoga videos, while Shiva Rea [www.shivarea.com] is known for mixing dance and yoga. John Friend [www.anusara.com] has trained thousands of teachers in his Anusara teaching methodology, and Wade Imre Morissette [www.wadeimremorissette.com] combines chanting with his teaching.

The good news is that you don't need to be a household name like the folks who grace the pages of *Yoga Journal*, but you do need to make some sort of a name for yourself. Coming up with creative ways to do that can be a fun and rewarding part of your work as a yoga teacher, and it can be a natural extension of the work you are doing in your hometown.

Teacher Marketing for the Wandering Yogi

It may sound a bit jaded, but you really can't count on other people—at least when it comes to marketing. A lot of yoga teachers think they can simply show up to teach a class at a local yoga studio or gym, and the masses will flock to them. This is not true for local teaching, and it is even less true when considering teaching outside your local community.

If you don't send press releases, develop high quality flyers, and post events to your website, as well as to other networking sites, there is a good chance the word won't get out. Remember, your big debut in a far off land may seem like the most important thing in the world to you, but to the studio owner, you are just another guest teacher. That is not to say they won't do their part, but with their busy schedules and full agendas, your event will not likely get the tender loving care that is needed to make it a success.

Studio Marketing

In spite of your best efforts, you will need the help of your host studio, as well as the teachers and staff at that studio! Keep in mind that most students in other cities won't know who you are. But when a teacher or front desk worker talks favorably about you, people listen.

While most yoga teachers and advanced yoga students know of Rodney Yee, most casual students wouldn't know who he is, beyond "That guy on all the yoga videos." If that is the case for Rodney Yee, just consider how much more likely it is for a teacher who hasn't been on Oprah's couch.

Consequently, it is essential that you get a clear commitment from the studio owner to promote your visit. Have the marketing details clearly spelled out in your contract, so that everyone is on board. Failure to do this will result in a tepid turnout at best.

Tip: Allow teachers and staff at the host studio to come to your workshop at a discount, or even for free, if space is available. People look to their teachers to know with whom they should study. Their opinion will carry more weight than any flyer you can put together. Even if you don't have a huge turnout for your first visit in a given city, you will be able to build a following among the leaders in that community, which will make marketing future events there much easier.

Travel and Expenses

When you travel and teach, there are expenses involved that don't apply when teaching in your hometown. Travel expenses such as airfare and hotels need to be factored into your budget. Consider this—it takes quite a few paying students just to cover the $400 flight and the $300 hotel room. And that is before you and the studio have even made any money on the event. Worse still, if you don't have enough paying students in your workshops, you can lose a lot of money.

Contract

Many yoga teachers like to go with the flow, and in many ways that is a good thing. But a lack of clarity in business relationships is not going with the flow. It's a recipe for an unmitigated disaster. This is where a contract comes in. It should spell out every detail of the event. Many of the larger studios may have a standard contract to sign, while others will expect you to draw one up. Here are a few key points to look for in a good contract.

A verbal contract isn't worth the paper it is written on.—Sam Goldwyn

Elements of a Good Contract

◊ Dates, times and locations

◊ Names of all people involved, including you, the studio, and the event's manager or studio owner

◊ Topics to be covered and the titles of the workshops

Financial agreement.

◊ Will you get paid a flat rate, a percentage of the money collected, or a percentage of the money after expenses?

◊ Will you require a minimum guarantee?

◊ When can you expect to be paid?

◊ Do you require a deposit?

Travel Logistics

◊ Where will you stay? If at a hotel, who will book the room?

◊ How will you get there? If plane, train, or bus, who will book the ticket?

Marketing:

◊ Who will send the press releases?

◊ Who will design and print the flyers?

◊ Will their staff be required to announce your workshop in their classes?

◊ What will you do to promote the event, such as send an email blast, post to your site, etc.?

Getting Paid

Every studio is different and every teacher has unique requirements. Senior teachers require a minimum turnout and a rather high financial guarantee. Lesser-known teachers usually have to make some concessions.

While I negotiate each contract separately, my standard agreement looks something like this:

70%-30% split after expenses

Minimum of $150 per workshop hour plus $50 per travel hour

While this may seem high, consider this. I spend hours flying across the country, teach for many hours, and then in my down time, I get to enjoy a sterile hotel room. I'm not complaining about this—I love traveling and teaching, but a tremendous amount of work beyond the actual teaching goes into being a wandering yogi. If you want to have a career that involves a lot of travel teaching, you need to factor in the toll it takes on your body, your social and family life, and the loss of income you incur from not teaching your regular classes while away from home.

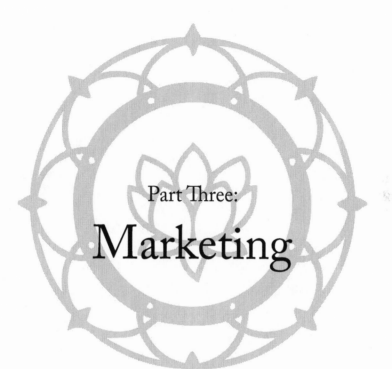

Part Three:
Marketing

Chapter 10:
A Yoga Teacher's Most Valuable Asset

Good teaching is one-fourth preparation and three-fourths pure theatre.
—*Gail Godwin*

What I'm about to tell you is perhaps the most important thing you can possibly learn from this book. It is the difference between becoming a mediocre yoga teacher and becoming an exceptional one. The reason people will want to take your class, or in some cases avoid your class, is because of you. To put a very fine point on it, your most valuable asset is YOURSELF.

I have two acquaintances who teach Bikram yoga and, in fact, both own their own studios. Unlike other forms of yoga, the Bikram practice is very standardized. Regardless of where you go in the world you will find the same sequence of twenty-six postures taught in a room that is 105° F. In theory, you could go to any Bikram teacher and expect the same experience. Yet my friend Lamott Atkins' [www.bikramyogacastro.com] class is full of loyal students—many of whom have been with him for years. Another acquaintance, whom I will call Bill, has trouble keeping a regular following.

Lamott cares deeply for his students and knows them all by name. He takes the time to listen to their concerns and needs, and remembers the details of their lives. Bill on the other hand, while skilled at teaching the Bikram sequence, is frequently in a bad mood and never asks students how they are doing. He frequently makes disparaging comments toward students in class and knows very few of their names. Bill remarked to me once that he couldn't understand why people flock to Lamott's studio rather than his own, even though his studio is more centrally located.

It doesn't matter if you are selling cars, pizza, soft drinks, or yoga; any good marketing expert will tell you that keeping the customers you already have is every bit as important as finding new ones. Good customer-service skills are essential for keeping the students you have, encouraging regular attendance, and building a sense of community. Your loyal students are your best marketers.

Think about your hairstylist, massage therapist, favorite books, and restaurants. Chances are that you have recommended them to your friends and family. This principle is true for yoga teachers as well. If you treat your students well, they will be one of your strongest marketing assets. Yet surprisingly few yoga teachers understand this basic principle.

Your greatest asset as a teacher is yourself!

The warmth and personality you bring to your classes is at the crux of what it means to be a successful yoga teacher. Teaching is so much more than telling someone how to execute a sequence of postures. To truly teach yoga, you need to learn to hold a safe space in which students can look deep within, and let go of long held blocks (samskaras) that prevent them from experiencing deep and lasting joy. Letting go of these energetic and psychic blocks is not an easy process and is often very scary. Consequently, your ability to guide them through the process from a place of compassion is essential if you truly want to succeed as a teacher.

There are a number of models for creating this safety but my personal favorite comes from motivational speaker and author, Dale Carnegie [www.dalecarnegie.com]. Although Carnegie died in 1955, his philosophy of working with people is timeless and particularly apt for yoga teachers. In his most well known book, *How to Win Friends and Influence People,* he lists a number of simple tools for holding space for the people in your life—be they friends, colleagues, or clients. I have found his techniques invaluable in my efforts to create a safe space for my students. In fact, I strongly encourage the participants in the Yoga Tree Teacher Training Program to read *How to Win Friends and Influence People* and even offer extra credit for doing so.

All the suggestions he offers for working with people are useful. I can't recommend the book highly enough, and several of his principles are particularly apt for yoga teachers. I would like to highlight a few of his key points.

Learn Your Students' Names

I don't remember anybody's name. How do you think the "dahling" thing got started?—Zsa Zsa Gabor

Many yoga teachers dread the thought of bumping into a yoga student outside of class, because they haven't taken the time to learn their students' names. This is unfortunate because it is one of the single most important things you can do. Many people will tell you they don't like their names, but all humans love the sound of their name when someone takes the time to remember it. When you remember students' names it tells them you care about them, that you value their presence in your class, and that they are not just another sweaty body in a sea of yogis.

If I were to tell you that I would pay you $500 to remember my name, you would commit it to memory for life. Now consider this: if I were to take your class twice a week for a year, and the studio where you work pays you $5 per head, that adds up to $500. Many of my students have been studying with me for ten or more years. This is in part because I'm a skilled yoga teacher, but the bigger reason they have stayed with me for so long is because they know I care about them.

Do I know every student by name? No, but I do make an effort. Even if I mistake someone named Mary for Maria or Jack for John, the effort alone is often enough to impress people, and if I forget a name completely, I'm never afraid to ask. To say, "I'm sorry, but could your remind me your name?" is another way of saying, "I value you enough to make the effort to learn."

Tip: When you meet someone, ask his or her name. Then during your conversation, repeat their name several times. If it is a common name, try to associate a facial feature with someone you know. For example, if I meet someone named Kathy, I look for a feature they share with my mother, who is also named Kathy. In this way, I have an instant clue. If they have a name that is not so common, I try to associate them with a famous person. For example, if a woman named Angelina takes your class and has big, pouty lips, you can easily associate her with Angelina Jolie. The only caution is to choose a feature that is not likely to change. Hairstyles, clothing, and even body shapes and sizes can change over time, whereas eye color, noses, lips, jaw lines, and the like tend to stay consistent over time.

Don't Criticize, Condemn, or Complain

Any fool can criticize, condemn and complain and most fools do.
—Benjamin Franklin

I once went to a class with a now former Yoga Tree teacher. After the class we were chatting, and every other word out of her mouth was critical. She was critical of the management at Yoga Tree and of the other teachers. She even complained about students—worse still, she did this within earshot of students.

While it may have been satisfying on some level for her to trash-talk others, it told me a few things about her. First, she was judgmental. I had a very clear sense that she would be complaining about me as soon as we were apart. Whether or not she did, I have no idea, but I was certainly left with the feeling that she would. Second, her condemnation of others did not make her seem more enlightened. In fact, she seemed petty and insecure. Third, it was clear that she had little interest in seeing the good in people—a fundamental quality of a successful teacher.

Not surprisingly, her classes were not well attended and she quit Yoga Tree in disappointment. What she failed to realize is that being overly critical and complaining is like white sugar. It may feel good in the moment, but it is rarely worth the crash that follows. Speaking your truth is very important, but there is a well-defined line between honestly expressing yourself in ethical dialog and complaining.

For example, if she had an issue with the Yoga Tree management, she could easily have called the owner and sat down for tea to express her concerns face-to-face. Furthermore, she could have expressed those concerns in a respectful way. Perhaps the management would have seen her point of view and made adjustments, or perhaps they would not have been willing or able to accommodate her requests. But one thing is certain; she would not have turned off students by complaining in front of them.

When students hear you complain or condemn, they will be naturally repelled even if you are talking about someone they don't know. The reverse is also true. If you can find the good in people and situations and talk about that, then you will draw people to you in droves.

Karl Erb [www.yoganexus.com], one of San Francisco's senior yoga teachers, was recently diagnosed with cancer. In addition to the cancer causing a host of health problems, he also had to endure aggressive chemotherapy and surgery. If anyone had the right to complain it was Karl, as life had certainly dealt him a difficult hand.

As Karl underwent his treatments he kept a blog that was honest, sincere, and even funny at times. When he was afraid or angry, he expressed that, but never in a complaining tone. He also continually expressed his gratitude for the support his students and fellow teachers were offering. In sharing so openly and honestly and never complaining, he inspired the San Francisco yoga community deeply. While he could have used his illness as an excuse to complain, he instead turned it into one of the greatest examples of yoga teaching I have ever witnessed.

Honest and Sincere Appreciation

Appreciation is a wonderful thing: It makes what is excellent in others belong to us as well.—Voltaire

In the Disney classic, Bambi we heard, "If you can't say something nice, don't say anything at all." On one level this is very good advice. On another level, it is only half the story. If you can't find something nice to say, then you haven't taken the time to look.

To pile false compliments on your students, however well intentioned, is little more than a lie. To do this may fool some people, but most will simply view you as insincere. To appreciate someone, you must do it from a place of honesty, and that can often mean taking the time to look.

I have an elderly student who takes my class at Grace Cathedral [www.labyrinthyoga.com]. His yoga poses often don't look like the poses the rest of the students are doing, and you won't be seeing him on the cover of *Yoga Journal* anytime soon. For me to say, "That is the best warrior pose ever!" would be a lie, and he would likely see right through it. But to say, "Good job! Your strength and balance are really improving!" would be entirely true, and the sincerity of my words would carry through.

To honestly appreciate your students' efforts on the yoga mat is one of the best ways to inspire them to feel welcome in your class and to continue to practice. Ask any grade school teacher about the effectiveness of giving stickers so students can proudly go home and hang their work on the refrigerator. We all need to have our efforts acknowledged, and if you can learn to do that in an honest and sincere way, students will flock to your classes and also develop a passion for their yoga practice.

Arouse an Eager Want

When a man is willing and eager the gods join in.—Aeschylus

People do yoga for all sorts of reasons, and the list of benefits a regular yoga practice can bestow are seemingly endless. Yet most new students have only the slightest inclination as to what yoga can do for their lives. Most people come to yoga with a single goal in mind. Perhaps they want to gain flexibility or address an injury. Some want to manage stress, while others want to deepen their spirituality. All of these goals are noble in and of themselves, and all are worthwhile. Yet seasoned yogis know that yoga is much more than any one of these benefits. As yoga teachers we are also keenly aware of the difference between a daily practice and a weekly practice.

Several years ago John came to my class to address his low back pain. While yoga is very effective at alleviating many forms of back pain, it is not as simple as taking a muscle relaxant or a pain killer. Yoga must be practiced regularly and consistently. John would come to class once a week, and after each class he did feel some relief from his pain, but the discomfort would always return.

After about a month of weekly classes, I pulled John aside to see how he was doing. I could tell that he was feeling marginally better, but he still hobbled into class each week in much the same condition. In effect, he was treading water with his pain.

My goal in talking to him was to get him to practice at least three times per week. So I started my conversation with him by asking him how his yoga practice was working for him. I then asked him if he would like to experience more lasting results. Of course his answer was an excited, "Yes!" I then proceeded to explain to him that a more regular practice would yield more lasting and dramatic benefits. I asked him if he would be willing to try an experiment by taking three classes in the next week to see how it felt. Naturally he agreed and currently takes class with me four or more times a week.

Now I could have demanded that he take my class more, or shamed him for only practicing once a week, but that probably would not have created the same level of commitment. By finding something that he naturally and eagerly wanted—less pain, and then explaining to him how he could achieve that goal, he became excited about a more regular practice. The result for him was indeed less pain; the result for me was a more eager, regular student.

Become Genuinely Interested in Others

You can make more friends in two months by becoming interested in other people than you can in two years by trying to get other people interested in you.—Dale Carnegie

About a month ago, a student named Heather took my class. I hadn't seen Heather in over a year. The last time I saw her, she was suffering from back pain caused from a misaligned sacroiliac joint. In addition to remembering her name, which surprised her, I was able to ask her how her back was feeling, and if the chiropractor I had referred her to was able to help.

The look on her face was one of shock. She couldn't believe I could recall such detail about her body when it had been so long since I'd seen her. But because I was able to remember the details she had shared with me, she felt that I had really heard her a year earlier, and also that I cared enough to remember. This level of concern and respect for students is good for your karma and good for your business. Not only is it responsible as a teacher to remember important details about your students' health, it is also a great way to create a space where students want to come back to your class.

Another way to impress your students is to remember details about their lives that they choose to share with you. Perhaps a student tells you the names of their children, or that they are getting married soon. Maybe they let you know that they were caring for a sick parent, or that they are considering a change in occupation. Whatever the details, asking about them the next time you seem them, or from time to time, is a great way to cultivate a welcoming atmosphere, and your students will naturally want to visit regularly.

The truth is that all of us think the details of our own health and lives are important. How often in life does someone ask you about your life, and then care enough to follow up, even if the details seem trivial? Sadly, many people don't even get that level of interest in their lives from their significant other.

After I remembered Heather's name and the details of her back pain, she began taking my class regularly again. In and of itself that was worth the small effort it took to remember her. Better still, she brought three friends with her to class over the past month—each one dealing with an issue of their own. She took the time to introduce them to me and to remind them that I was the best teacher for them because of how much I was able to help her. In truth, what worked was not so much that I had helped her as much as I showed an interest in something that was naturally very important to her—her own health and wellbeing.

Smile

> Smile. Have you ever noticed how easily puppies make
> human friends? Yet all they do is wag their tails and fall
> over.—Walter Anderson, The Confidence Course

The next time you are holding a baby, try this experiment. Offer them a beaming smile, and see what happens. They will reflexively smile back. Of course the opposite is true as well. If you hand that infant to someone who habitually frowns, the baby will instinctively reject the person and might even start to cry.

While we might develop the ability to hide our reactions to both smiles and scowls, we never outgrow the internal reaction that the facial expression of another evokes within us. When your students enter your class and see a teacher who is smiling, they will automatically feel at ease. Even before the first downward dog, they have started to soften and let down their guard.

There is one important thing to remember, however. The smile must be genuine. If you are faking your smile, you may well come off as a serial killer rather than a compassionate yoga teacher. Of course, some days smiling honestly is easier than others. This is where the practice of gratitude can be very helpful. If you can find something you are genuinely grateful for, however small, you will smile sincerely. If, however, you are simply flashing a toothy grin to hide the bad day you're having, you will simply amplify the negativity you are bringing into the yoga class.

Be a Good Listener

Listen to many, speak to a few.—William Shakespeare

What do hairstylists, bartenders, and yoga teachers have in common? People tell all three very personal details of their lives. My Aunt Josie was a hair stylist for years and often knew when her clients were getting a divorce before their husbands did. Yet she was very clear about not repeating the details of her clients' lives, because she knew that her clients trusted her. She understood that the reasons women came to her salon had at least as much to do with her ability to listen as it did with the haircut she was offering.

It's important to note that your job as a yoga teacher is first and foremost to listen. When you assume the role of teacher, you are making an agreement to place your needs to the side and to find other ways to get those needs met. Just as a parent must listen to a child's hopes, fears, and concerns with infinite patience, we as yoga teachers need to offer our students the same level of care if we want to create a space where people can journey deep into themselves.

We live in a world where people can go for days or weeks without anyone taking the time to listen to them. Coworkers, acquaintances and even friends and family can get so busy or self-absorbed that they can forget to listen. We all need to be heard. If you can take the time to listen to your students—really listen—you will earn their trust. And if you can remember the details of what they shared with you the next time they come to your class, and then check in with them, they will know that you care, and that you value their presence in your life.

People are hungry for a compassionate ear that isn't hard-wired to the mouth. If someone tells you something in confidence, honor that. It may be something about their body, their emotional or psychological life, or something seemingly unrelated to yoga. By refraining from blabbing the details of their lives to others (including your romantic partner), you build an environment of trust and safety. Even the students who choose not to share personal details, will feel that aura of safety and will visit your class often. We are all hungry for a safe place in this often cruel world. If you can provide that space, students will yearn to take your class—the catch is that you have to earn and maintain their trust first. Don't expect it to be given to you freely, and remember—you will not likely regain that trust if you abuse it!

Discuss Their Interests and Issues

Taking an interest in what others are thinking and doing is often a much more powerful form of encouragement than praise.—Robert Martin

I have a confession. I hate watching sports on TV. My personal interest in sports in which I'm not a participant is actually less than zero. That said, if you come to my class and share with me that you are excited about the World Series being on TV, then that is what we will talk about. Not only that, the next time I see you in class, I will ask you if the team you were rooting for came out on top.

Take a moment and think about the things that interest you. Some might be insignificant or silly even. Maybe you are really into Star Trek or perhaps you like fly-fishing. Other things may be more significant to you—your work, romantic partner, or your children. Regardless of how big or small those things are in your life, they are important to you, and that is what you most enjoy talking about.

Your students are not different from you. While their personal interests may differ from yours, they are most happy when they are talking about the things they feel most passionate about. If you want your students to leave your class feeling good about their time with you, then let them lead the conversation. Talk about their kids or their hobbies, and find something about what they are saying that can excite you as well.

For example, if you wanted to talk about the World Series, I could mention an article about a famous baseball player or coach that incorporates yoga into their training. There is almost no topic in which you cannot find common ground with another person.

Tip: Always talk about what your students want to discuss, and then find a way to share in their excitement on that subject.

Avoid Arguments

Anger is never without an argument, but seldom with a good one.
—Indira Gandhi

It is conventional wisdom that you should never discuss religion or politics in polite company, and yet you would be surprised how many students and yoga teachers didn't get that memo. Like most people you probably have passionate views on a whole range of subjects, and chances are some of your students will have different opinions.

Several years ago there was a woman who took my class regularly. Although she no longer attended synagogue she still felt many bonds with the Jewish community. When she found out that she was pregnant and that she was going to have a son, she was torn. On the one hand circumcision is an important rite for Jews. On the other hand she had been receiving a lot of pressure from her husband and non-Jewish friends to forego what they viewed as a barbaric ritual of genital mutilation.

As she shared this personal dilemma with me, I could feel emotions building within me, as I have strong feelings on the subject. But my opinion would not likely change her mind, and it could only serve to add to the anxiety she was feeling. Although the pull was strong for me to give her my heavy-handed views on the subject, I knew better and resisted the urge.

What resulted was magical. Because she had been pushed and pulled by all the people in her life to choose one option or the other, she viewed my simple listening as a refuge, and by extension my classes as well. Having an opinion is easy, and most people delight in arguing their point of view as if it were the only point of view in the room. If you can resist the urge to argue—and it may be quite strong, you will find that people will soften around you and will feel welcome in your class.

Admit When You Are Wrong

If you are willing to admit your faults, you have one less fault to admit.
—Unknown

I have a very dry sense of humor, which some people love and others are deeply offended by. Several years ago I was teaching a class on Gay Pride day. At the start of the class I made a comment, which I intended to be humorous. "I want to thank all of the straight people who came to class today and ventured through all the Gay Pride traffic. I would also like to thank the gay people who came this morning for not having any pride—it is great to have you all here."

Most people chuckled knowing that I am gay myself. Yet after class a young man came up to me and was visibly upset. He explained that he was gay, and that he had made a very conscious choice to attend my class as a way of celebrating his growth around self-acceptance. As a teen he lived under a constant cloud of self-loathing because of his sexuality, but through many years of personal work, he had learned to love himself. Because yoga had been so instrumental in his healing, he wanted to start his Gay Pride celebration with a yoga class.

My ego immediately reacted with a surge of defensiveness, and for a moment I considered debating the merits of what I had said. Rather than defend my comments, however, I simply apologized. "I am so sorry about my comment. I can see where that must have sounded very insensitive."

He immediately softened, and we proceeded to have a very sweet and uplifting conversation. Happily, he is a regular student to this day. Had I held the defensive posture that my ego was in favor of, I likely would have turned him off and would never have seen him again. What's worse, he might have discouraged others from taking my class as well. The simple act of admitting a mistake created a relationship of healing rather than conflict—which, of course, is what yoga is all about.

Discuss Your Own Faults and Failings First

Many teachers make the mistake of teaching only the poses they do best. Some of the poses at which I am most skilled at teaching, however, are not poses that I have personally perfected. In fact, sometimes it's just the opposite. Frequently, when I am going to demonstrate a pose, I point out the areas of that pose where I still struggle. This gives my students permission to struggle with their poses, because they can clearly see there is no shame in the struggle. A true yogi is one who embraces the stumbling and falling, the shaking and sweat, the tight tendons, and the weak abs. This is not to say that we don't strive to build strength, flexibility and dexterity—it simply means we meet ourselves where the body is, rather than where the ego thinks it should be.

The same is true of the relationships we form with our students. Some teachers falsely believe that they can never show their students any disturbance in their piece of mind. This is very unfortunate for several reasons.

First it is wholly unrealistic. We all have upsets, and to pretend otherwise is dishonest. This charade can only be maintained for so long, and when your students see a crack in the façade, they will resent you for the lie. The only thing people love to do more than put someone on a pedestal, is to see them fall off.

Second, you set up unrealistic expectations for your students. Yoga is not about never getting upset. It is about weathering that upset in a more enlightened way. To the degree that your students are able to see you manage your upsets—big or small, in a more yogic way, is the degree to which they will learn to do the same.

Third, each time you stumble and fall, and pick yourself up again, others will realize their own power. When I was in the sixth grade, my teachers convinced my mother that it would be best if I repeated the year. I was filled with guilt and shame as my friends and classmates went on to the seventh grade without me. At the time I was an altar boy at Saint Michael's church. Although I usually tuned out the sermons, I clearly remember one that gave me the strength to move forward.

The sermon concerned the Gospel narrative in which Jesus fell under the weight of his cross three times. The priest explained that Jesus falling was not a sign of weakness, but that each time he got up was a sign of strength. He went on to remind everyone that Jesus continuing to get up again under such extreme circumstances showed great strength. He explained that each of us could do the same in the face of much less daunting trials.

Somehow that sermon struck a chord deep within me and I was able to face the challenges in front of me. More importantly, it taught me that, as a teacher, showing my faults and failings was not a weakness but rather a strength.

When we show our vulnerabilities, we empower our students to embrace theirs. There is no shame in falling out of a pose or coming to child's pose on the mat, nor should there be any shame when we stumble and fall in life. In fact there are few things more empowering than embracing our weaknesses.

The world-renowned American mystic, Swami Chetananda [www.chetananda.org] once said, "Pain is your best friend. It is infinitely more honest with you than pleasure. Despite what you might think, the painful experiences you have benefit you far more than the pleasurable ones, even though most of us spend our lives trying to duck and hide from them. But when you can center yourself and be open to look pain in the eye, you have transcended the limits of your ego and this humanity. It is then that you enter into the possibility of becoming a great being."

Praise Every Improvement

A pat on the back is only a few vertebrae removed from a kick in the pants, but is miles ahead in results.—Ella Wheeler Wilcox

As a child, I loved to come home from school with sticker or a star on my paper so that my mom could post it prominently on the refrigerator and then boast about my achievements to my father when he came home from work. We all love to have our achievements praised and acknowledged as children, and that need never goes away.

There is a delightful woman named Doris who takes my class at Grace Cathedral every week. Though she is well into her senior years, she has refused to tell me exactly how old she is. She recently moved to San Francisco to live with her daughter due to her deteriorating vision.

Because of her vision loss, balance is exceedingly difficult for her, so when I teach tree pose, I frequently offer her my arm as a support. At first she struggled, even with my help, but over several weeks, I noticed that she was using my arm less and less. Though her execution of tree pose was very modified, she was improving each week.

"Doris," I said, "That is amazing! Your balance is improving so fast! Can you feel the difference?" She beamed with pride in much the same way I did in the second grade when my work was acknowledged.

So I asked her if she would like to improve even more. She was enthusiastic. I instructed her to stand near a wall or counter at home a few times every day to practice tree. She could use the wall or counter as much as needed, but she could also practice taking her hand away as much as her balance would allow.

Doris comes to my class faithfully every week and is sure to show me how much she has improved. The simple act of praising her efforts inspired her to start a home practice and to get really excited about her yoga.

Every last one of your students is like Doris. If you give your students honest and sincere praise and acknowledge their achievements—no matter how small those achievements might be—you will inspire them to work harder, become more disciplined, and, of course, attend your class with greater regularity.

Give them a Reputation to Live Up To

A master can tell you what he expects of you. A teacher, though, awakens your own expectations.—Patricia Neal

If you tell a child he is stupid over and over again, he will believe it, and his school grades will suffer. His self esteem will stagnate, and the prospects for that child excelling in life will be greatly diminished. Likewise, if you affirm a child as smart over and over again, that child will likely do well in school, have a healthy self-esteem and a much greater chance of success in life.

Psychologists refer to this principle as a self-fulfilling prophecy. What's more, it's not just children who are susceptible to a self-fulfilling prophecy. All of us are more likely to live up to our reputations, and this is even more the case when an authority figure such as a teacher, counselor, or mentor offers a vision of who we are and who we could be.

Handstand is a very powerful pose, and yet very few people believe they can do it. The other day I had a woman in my class who simply sat on her mat sulking when I asked everyone to go to the wall. I went over to her to see what was wrong and in a sullen voice she said, "I can't do this pose."

"Yet." I said.

"Excuse me?" she replied.

"You can't do this pose yet!" I said. "Believe me when I tell you, you are strong enough and have the balance required to do this pose, and if you let me work with you, I think you will surprise yourself."

"Well, what do you want me to do?" she asked skeptically.

"For today, I simply want you to move your mat to the wall, place your hands about six inches from the wall and hop your leg up three or four times. I don't want you to kick all the way up today. Just hop a little higher each time."

"Well, I guess I could do that," she said.

A few things followed that are worth noting. First, she was no longer sitting on her mat doing nothing and feeling sorry for herself. Rather than sulking and comparing herself to the other students, she was moving forward. Second, she began to smile and that smile remained on her face as she left the class. And third, the next time she came to class she asked if we could work on handstands again—and this time she was able to kick all the way up to the wall with my help. She left the class with a bounce in her step that I had never seen before.

Our primary objective as teachers is to see in our students the potential that they can't yet see in themselves—then to empower them, guide them, and support them in reaching those potentials. When we give a student a reputation to live up to, we empower them to find the inner strength and fortitude that can move mountains in their lives.

This not only applies to the yoga poses we teach. I had a student stay after class a few months ago who had broken down in class. He was embarrassed by his emotional outburst and wanted to apologize. I assured him that emotional release was a natural part of the practice and then asked him what was going on in his life.

"In the span of two months, I have lost my job, and my wife left me. Sometimes I don't think I have what it takes to even get out of bed in the morning." His eyes began to well up again.

"And yet here you stand. You did get out of bed today, and not only that, you managed to come to a yoga class, which is more than most people in your situation would be able to do. I can only imagine what you must be feeling right now, but I have to say, I'm inspired by your strength. It is because of that strength that I know you will come out the other side," I responded.

He looked genuinely surprised by my comments, but his face softened and he straightened his back. He gave me a big hug and left with a bit more energy than he came in with.

I wasn't just telling him he was strong. In my perception he was very strong, and in my telling him the truth as I saw it, he left with a reputation to live up to. In the months that followed, he began attending class daily and recently told me that he had decided to enroll in the Yoga Teacher Training at Yoga Tree.

"Man, Shiva[1] has kicked my ass!" he told me. "But you know what? I'm grateful, because I feel like a new chapter in my life is beginning! I feel stronger and more hopeful than ever before in my life!"

---

1   Shiva is the Hindu deity associated with transformation, destruction and rebirth.

Your Strongest Asset

In the next chapter we will explore a number of marketing techniques designed to invite people into your class, but the thing to remember is that all of your marketing efforts will be in vain if you don't create a space where your students feel empowered, cared for, and important.

Your students are both your livelihood and your greatest source of inspiration. If you treat them well and provide a space in which they can heal their bodies, quiet their minds, and take bold steps along the spiritual path, they will find refuge in your classes. This is good for them and good for your business.

> *People are often unreasonable, illogical, and self-centered;*
> *forgive them anyway.*
> *If you are kind, people may accuse you of selfish, ulterior motives;*
> *Be kind anyway.*
> *If you are successful, you will win some false friends and some true*
> *enemies; succeed anyway.*
> *If you are honest and frank, people may cheat you;*
> *Be honest and frank anyway.*
> *What you spend years building, someone could destroy overnight;*
> *Build anyway.*
> *If you find serenity and happiness, there may be jealousy;*
> *be happy anyway.*
> *The good you do today, people will often forget tomorrow;*
> *Do good anyway.*
> *Give the world the best you have, and it may never be enough;*
> *Give the world the best you've got anyway.*
> *You see, in the final analysis, it is between you and God;*
> *it was never between you and them anyway.*
> — *Mother Theresa*

Chapter 11:
Marketing on a Budget

How people treat you is their karma; how you react is yours.
—Wayne Dyer

Is Good Marketing Good Karma

It seems like every time you turn on the TV, listen to the radio, or pick up the newspaper you are bombarded with advertisements that are misleading and unethical. Most marketing campaigns are designed to make you feel less-than, in order to convince you that you need a given product or service to make you whole.

Obviously these marketing campaigns must work, or the companies that are spending billions on these campaigns would not be doing it; however, just because something is effective doesn't make it ethical. Aside from being unethical, there is an additional problem with this strategy—cost. It is extremely expensive to manufacture a false need so that people will want to buy your beer, makeup, cola, or car.

As yoga teachers we need to be ever mindful of our ethical obligations when marketing. The good news is there is an ethical way to market, and it is much more cost effective. In fact, many marketing techniques I will be discussing are both free and 100% ethical.

Why, you might ask, do large companies spend so much money on marketing, when much of what we can do as yoga teachers is free or low cost? Simply put, the need for yoga already exists. We don't have to manufacture a false need the way a company selling a sugary soft drink might, so our marketing costs are small in comparison.

Whether people want to improve their health, deepen their spirituality or reduce stress, yoga is a great way to fill those needs. You don't need to lie or mislead to sell yoga—you simply need to invite people to take your class. To deceive, manipulate, and give high-pressure sales pitches actually has the opposite effect when the need already exists. Thus, you simply need to reach out to potential students in ways that are creative and inspiring. In other words, good karma is good marketing!

You can be the best yoga teacher in the world, but if you don't market yourself, no one will know. Most of us don't like to market ourselves—it's just not in our nature. But if you really want to succeed as a yoga teacher it is absolutely essential.

San Francisco's largest yoga studio, Yoga Tree, has an enormous marketing effort, and that certainly helps all the teachers who work there. However, the teachers who really succeed are the ones who have their own marketing strategy, and implement it with as much vigor as they do their classes.

The important thing to remember is that marketing doesn't need to be expensive. Small marketing tasks done consistently will reap far greater rewards than that high-priced newspaper ad.

In the following pages I will be offering many free and low-cost things you can do to market yourself. You don't have to do every one, but doing something each day is the key.

Tip: For every hour you spend teaching, you should be spending an hour on your marketing efforts. Anything less will produce lackluster results.

Define Your Product

Look at any product or service on the market and you will see something very unique being presented. Even products with seemingly few differences are marketed in ways that aim to distinguish them from their competitors.

Take, for example, Coke and Pepsi. Both are colas and both taste roughly the same, but when you see an ad for one or the other, they both try to burn into your mind certain qualities that make their product unique, while beverages like 7-Up seek to carve out a niche as the "uncola."

As a yoga teacher you are a unique entity. Your life experiences, your talents and skills, and your personality bring to your class a one-of-a-kind experience that no one else can duplicate.

Maybe you are a psychologist, social worker, or a massage therapist, and those skills can dovetail with your work as a yoga teacher. Or maybe you have 'school of life' training that makes you more uniquely suited to work with certain types of students. Jeremi McManus [www.jeremimcmanus. com], for example, fuses his work as a psychotherapist with his yoga classes. This sets him apart. In addition to his professional training, Jeremi has a lot of life experience as a man who struggled at times to celebrate his masculinity and his spirituality in a culture that seems to pit these two aspects of his being against each other. Thus, Jeremi teaches yoga classes and facilitates relationship groups that create the space for this dilemma and others to be mindfully explored.

Become an Expert and Market Yourself Online

Because of your yoga training, you have a lot of information to share with the world, and the Internet is a great place to do it. There are numerous blogs, web magazines, and other outlets that are looking for content. Most won't pay you, but they will add a link to your website, and sometimes a photo of you next to the article. Some will even pay you a small stipend for your contribution. The most important thing is that you are getting your name and face out there and branding yourself as an expert in your field.

For example, if you work with the autoimmune disease, lupus, you could write a short web article entitled, "Five Ways Yoga Helps You Live with Lupus." By posting such articles you become the expert, and people living with lupus, as well as the doctors who treat it will know where to go.

Tip: Once your article is live on one website, you can email relevant blogs so they can post a link to the article. Since there are blogs for just about every subject imaginable, you can reach out to very targeted groups quite easily. For example, the article on Lupus we used as an example would likely be of great interest to the Lupus Yahoo and Facebook group, as well as the Lupus support page.

You are never given a wish without also being given the power to make it true. You may have to work for it, however.—Richard Bach

Long Haul Marketing

I worked at a yoga studio in San Francisco for a short time where the owner believed that simply running an ad or two in the SF Weekly Newspaper would bring a flood of people in the door. He spent a small fortune to have a fancy ad designed and ran the spot for one week. He was very disappointed when only two people showed up.

Effective marketing requires a plan and a sustained effort. In much the same way that you need to keep your heart rate up for a sustained period of time in order to get the benefits of cardiovascular exercise, you need to come up with a marketing plan and stick to it for an extended period of time. In fact, conventional marketing wisdom holds that it takes between six and twelve impressions before someone buys a good or a service.

In other words a potential student needs to hear about your class at least six times before he or she will decide to try your class. Now, not all impressions need to come from the same source. Perhaps they hear you interviewed on the radio, and then see your class reviewed on Yelp. Then they come across your website. Then they see a postcard of yours at the local café, notice your name listed on the schedule at the gym, and finally a friend tells them about your class. Likewise, not all of these impressions need to happen over a short period of time. This can take months or years.

In short, you need to keep your efforts sustained over time. You will also find that taking a multifaceted marketing approach that keeps your name and your brand out there in as many ways as possible will exponentially multiply your marketing efforts. You are far better off to do a number of the free or low cost techniques on the following pages than to spend a huge sum of money on one print ad that only appears in your local paper once. Consistency and longevity will trump big, flashy, and short-lived ads any day!

Customer Service

Courteous treatment will make a customer a walking advertisement.
—*James Cash Penney*

Reply to Emails

Free

Just before my first book, *Spiritual Journeys along the Yellow Brick Road*, came out, I spoke with a friend who had authored a number of books himself. It was an exciting time for me, and I could barely imagine what it would be like to have my words being read by complete strangers. I was both excited by the prospect and terrified that once I put my words out there, I would be judged. In many ways I felt like a mother watching her child venture out into the world on their own for the first time.

So in the midst of all this excitement and fear, I asked my friend what advice he had for me. His advice was so completely unexpected that I almost needed to sit down. "Write back to everyone who writes you," he proclaimed. "You won't be able to write volumes to each person, but write back to everyone without exception, even if it is just a sentence saying thank you for taking the time to write." That advice has turned out to be some of the most valuable and sound advice I have ever received!

There are three basic types of email you will receive in your inbox. The first is what I call "the inquiry" email. This type of email asks you questions about your schedule or teaching style, or perhaps if your class is appropriate for their particular needs. We live in a fast-paced world and the speed with which you reply to an inquiry email could very well determine whether that person decides to attend your class. In some cases, the email may come from an existing student asking about a new injury or another concern. Nothing says, "I care about your welfare," like a prompt reply.

The second type of email is what I call "Fan Mail." In this type of email, students will write to tell you how much they appreciate your class or about a particular success they have had. Nothing makes my day more than getting one of these emails. It adds wind to my sails.

There is a saying, "Only God knows how many apples are in an apple seed." As yoga teachers we are in the business of planting seeds. Some of those seeds will develop before our eyes, and that's a tremendous honor to witness. But more often than not, people will come to your class, experience healing and transformation, and then go about their lives. So we need to operate on faith that what we're doing is making a difference in the world.

When you receive an email from a student who thinks enough of your work to take the time to write, be sure to thank them. Then save that email for a day when you really need a boost. It doesn't matter how busy I am, I always make time to drop a short thank you reply, because without the occasional positive feedback, it would be impossible for me to do the work I do.

There will be days when you don't think you have what it takes to stand in front of a room and lead yet another round of sun salutations. When those days come around, open your "fan mail" folder and reread a gratitude letter.

The third type is the most difficult type of email. It is what I call, "Attack Mail." In this type of email you can expect some harsh words. Since the internet affords some anonymity, many people feel free to let you have it. Sometimes their concerns are legitimate, while other times they may simply need to vent. In either case, it is very important to respond in a kind and courteous manner.

It is so natural to want to strike back when someone attacks you, and yet no good can come of that. When my fourth book, *Hearts & Minds: Talking to Christians about Homosexuality*, was released, I received a flood of email. Given the controversial nature of the book, much of it was hostile. Take the following exchange, for example.

Dear Mr. Main,

I read about your book on the internet and I felt moved to write you. The Bible is very clear on the subject of homosexuality. There is nothing to talk about. Either you believe the Bible or you believe the homosexual agenda. I fear for your soul and I hope that you will find Jesus before it is too late.

In Christ's Love,

Celia

Celia,

Thank you so much for taking the time to write. You clearly have strong feelings about this subject, and I'm honored that you thought enough of my work to share your views. I know this is a very difficult subject and like you, I have given it a lot of thought. While you and I may disagree on many things, I appreciate your being kind and polite.

In my book I make a case for why I believe that homosexuality and the Bible are not necessarily in conflict. I would love to send you a copy of my book. If you would be so kind, I would appreciate your looking it over and alerting me to any factual errors you may come across. My goal is to represent the Bible and Christians in a fair and honest light, while at the same time conveying my own views on the subject. Your input would be very welcome.

Sincerely,

Darren

Celia and I exchanged a few more emails after that, and I did send her my book. She even asked my advice in reaching out to her gay nephew from whom she had been estranged for a number of years. Had I responded to Celia in a reactionary way, I would have no doubt validated her suspicion that I was a sinner. She would not have stopped to reconsider her views, and it may have been many more years before she reached out to her nephew.

When we receive criticism about our work, it is best to take a few deep breaths before responding. In many cases, disgruntled people simply want to be heard. When you allow them to vent, they will soften their stance and may even return to your class. Others may want to pick a fight, and I can assure you that it is a fight you will never win, because even if you succeed in proving them wrong, they will still think ill of you.

There is a story from India in which a wealthy businessman had two sons. His youngest son heard Gautama, the Buddha, speak and was so enchanted that he left home to follow the master. The father sent his oldest son to fetch his younger brother, but when he found him, he had the occasion to hear the great teacher speak. He too was so inspired that he did not return home either.

The father was irate for he had lost both sons to the Buddha. There was no one to take over the family business and no one to care for him and his wife in their old age. So he went to the teacher to give him a piece of his mind. When he finally found Gautama, he screamed and yelled until he ran out of breath, and then screamed some more. The great one looked on the man calmly with compassion in his eyes and when the man had released all of his fury, the Buddha quietly asked him, "If you buy your wife a gift and offer it to her, and she refuses to accept it, what becomes of the gift?"

The man was perplexed by this odd question, but answered, "I suppose the gift would remain with me."

"That is correct," the Buddha said calmly. "I do not accept your gift of anger, but if you allow me, I will teach you to meditate so you can no longer be angry." The man bowed at the teacher's feet and asked him humbly if he and his wife could join him.

When we respond to criticism in a dignified and kind way, we not only refuse to accept their 'gift of anger,' but we also invite them to look at that anger and perhaps find a better way to dissolve it.

Send Thank You Cards

Free

At the risk of sounding like Miss Manners, be sure to send thank you notes to anyone and everyone who supports you—whether it's your doctor, your accountant, the student who brought a friend to class, or the manager who interviewed you for a potential job. If another professional refers a student to your class or a fellow teacher tips you off about a job opening, send a note. For the cost of a postage stamp, you can let them know you are grateful for their support!

We all get a lot of mail, the lion's share of which is bills and junk mail. It's always a welcome relief to receive a note of acknowledgement. Such a simple gesture can result in more referrals in the future. Sadly, it is a dying art, but that will make your note stand out even more!

Tips:
◊ Always handwrite the note.
◊ It can be short and sweet.
◊ When appropriate, invite them to take a class as your guest.
◊ Offer to support them in some way

Sample Thank You note

Doctor Johnson,

Thanks so much for seeing me on such short notice. I know you are busy, so I was very grateful that you were able to arrange your schedule to accommodate me. It is nice to know I have a doctor who is there for me when I need him. That is so hard to find, and your kindness made my healing that much easier.

Sincerely,

Darren
PS: If you ever want to take a yoga class, I would love to offer you a class as my guest. It is the least I can do.

Befriend Front Desk Staff

Free

Whether you work at a gym or a yoga studio, be sure to learn the names of the front desk staff. Welcome them into your classes, and always thank them for helping you out. The front desk staff make up the face of that studio or gym, and when people stop in looking for a good yoga class, who do you think will come to mind? Will it be the person who is kind to them, remembers their name, and welcomes them to take his or her yoga class? Or will it be the person who all but ignores them?

Sadly a lot of teachers don't bother to say hello to the front desk workers and treat their presence in class as a burden. I will never understand this, as a huge percentage of the referrals to my classes come from the front desk. In truth, the front desk staff are among your best assets, and the fact that they work so hard to support you, combined with their ability to help in marketing your class, make them among the most important people in your professional life.

Birthday Class Free

Free

Some people like to make a big deal out of their birthdays, while others would rather forego the cake and confetti. But almost everyone likes getting gifts. If you know one of your students is celebrating a birthday, invite him or her to take a class as your guest. Better yet, make it known on your website and flyers that everyone gets a free class during their birthday week.

This policy is simple, it costs you nothing, and it has four very tangible benefits. First, it makes your students feel special. Second, it will inspire students who have not taken your class in a while to return. Third, it may give a student who has not yet tried your class the nudge they need to check you out. Fourth, birthdays are a great time to reflect on the past and to make commitments and resolutions for the year to come. Your offering them a free class to help celebrate their special day may remind them of just how important yoga is to their health and well-being and thus, your classes are likely to be part of their birthday resolutions.

First Class Free

Free

Assuming the studio or gym you work for is open to it, make it known on your website and on your printed schedule, that the first class is always free for new students. If a student tries your class and likes it, you may have a regular student for years to come. True, some students will not come back or will take advantage, but on the whole, I have found this to be a very effective way to build my classes quickly and to develop a large following of students. The vast majority of people who try your class are likely to feel the benefits of yoga and return.

If you get their email address, send them a follow up email thanking them for taking your class and check in to see how they felt in the days that followed. This is a great way to let them know you care, while at the same time reminding them about the experience they had both in your class and with the post class bliss that most new students feel.

Complimentary Class

Free

The other day, a student came into Yoga Tree to take my class. She had walked several blocks in the cold January rain and, believing she had pre-paid classes in the system, she left her wallet at home. Unfortunately this student had used up all of her classes and was going to be turned away.

Overhearing the conversation I interrupted. "You can allow her in as my guest." Although she was a student I had never worked with, it didn't feel right to send her out into a rainstorm. I had no ulterior motives; it just seemed like the right thing to do.

What was interesting was that that simple act of kindness, which cost me absolutely nothing, had very wide reaching effects. One gentleman approached me after class saying, "I overheard what you did for the woman who left her wallet at home, and it's nice to know that yoga isn't always business as usual. You will be seeing a lot more of me."

A few days later, the same woman returned to my class and even purchased two of my books, asking me to sign one for her and one for her daughter. As I was signing the books, she said, "You don't know how much that meant to me the other day. I had learned that my daughter had a miscarriage earlier that day. She lives in Europe and I was feeling so overwhelmed and helpless. I don't think I have ever needed a yoga class as much as I did that day! I want to be there for my daughter, but given the distance it is just not practical, so I'm going to send her your book in hopes it will give her some clarity in this difficult time."

So one simple free class resulted in at least two loyal students and the sale of two books. Of course, I didn't have all that in mind when I allowed her to be my guest, but a simple offering like that can branch out in ways that are impossible to imagine. It is for this reason that I give away free classes like candy on Halloween. Here are a few examples:

◊ If someone has an injury or medical concern that might be improved with yoga.

◊ If you know someone is having a hard time financially.

◊ As part of a thank you note.

◊ When you meet someone on the street, at a party or other gathering who expresses an interest in yoga.

◊ If someone has a friend or family member in town, offer to comp their guest.

Reward Referrals

Free

You may not know it, but you have a virtual army of people who would love to spread the word about your classes. They are your students, and their efforts to bring their friends and family to your class will be one of the most amazing ways you can market yourself.

Some teachers and studios set up a referral program in which students can earn free classes for each friend they bring. This can be very effective, but it can easily feel like a Ponzi scheme. I prefer a more subtle approach. When a student has referred a few students to my class, I either pull them aside to express my gratitude, or I send them a thank you note. I also ask them to take their next class as my guest.

However you decide to reward referrals, know that it will generate even more good will and will encourage your students to continue to recommend you to their circle of friends.

Invite Feedback

Free

If a student compliments you on your class you should do two things immediately.

First, thank them. Humbly receive their gratitude! Second, ask them if they would be willing to fill out a comment card (assuming the studio offers the cards) or barring that, ask them to email the management. Most students are thrilled to do that, and nothing will get you more classes in better time slots like emails from students who have enjoyed your class.

It is important that you not be pushy, and ask from a place of humility, or you may evoke their ire, and the management may be getting a very different email than the one you had hoped for!

Networking

> *The successful networkers I know, the ones receiving tons of referrals and feeling truly happy about themselves, continually put the other person's needs ahead of their own.—Bob Burg*

The Elevator Pitch

When I first started getting phone calls from radio stations wanting to interview me about my work I was very excited, but I had a very difficult lesson to learn. Given the nature of broadcast media, I always felt like I could barely get a sentence or two out before the host would cut me off to move on to the next segment.

My publicist counseled me on what is called in publicity circles, "The Elevator Pitch." The idea is simple. You need to get your pitch down to the length of time it would take you to sell your book, CD, yoga class, or whatever else, in the time it takes to ride in an elevator with someone.

Most people are busy and even in social settings such as a cocktail party, they will not want to give you a lot of their time. Therefore, you need to have your pitch down to a few sentences that will inspire them to want more information from you.

Take a moment to practice right now. Imagine you just got into an elevator only to find Oprah Winfrey is standing next to you. She smiles and asks you why she should come to your yoga class. What do you say?

If you find this exercise difficult, it is not surprising, but it is extremely valuable to refine how you would respond. Now the chance of your sharing an elevator with Oprah Winfrey is slim, but the principle is the same if you are talking to a stranger on the bus, another professional, or someone who calls you looking for more information about your classes. The more prepared you are to answer these questions, the better you will be at sounding like you are a teacher worth having.

It is also helpful to write out twenty questions and answers that are likely to be asked of you, along with your responses. You don't need to memorize the answers word for word, but having thought about the questions before you are asked them will help prevent the "deer caught in headlights" look.

Sample Questions

◊ Why should I do yoga?

◊ I'm not very flexible. Can I still do yoga?

◊ I have an injury. Is it safe for me to do yoga?

◊ Is yoga a religious cult?

◊ What style of yoga do you teach?

◊ Do you teach yoga in a hot room?

◊ Do you work with beginners?

◊ Will I be the oldest/youngest person in the room?

Assist Senior Yoga Teachers

Free

Stephanie Snyder [www.stephaniesnyder.com], one of San Francisco's most popular yoga teachers, wasn't always a rock star in the yoga world. Like every one else, she started as a student and then completed her first teacher training. At first things started off slow for her, but within a few years, her classes grew precipitously until there was a wait-list to get in the door. In addition to being a very skilled teacher she has always considered herself a student first and a teacher second. One thing Stephanie did a lot when she first started teaching was to assist senior yoga teachers. She did this for her own growth and development, but it had the added benefit of introducing her to large numbers of students. Many students who had not heard the name Stephanie Snyder quickly became aware of her, and when they saw her name appearing on studio schedules, there was an established rapport.

One of the fastest ways to build your reputation, continue your education and open doors in your local community is to find a senior yoga teacher to assist.

Sub, Sub, and Sub Some More!

Earns You Money

Once I was preparing to sub for a popular teacher at Yoga Tree. I was sitting off to the side scanning through a book of quotes looking for a meditation with which to open the class. It was then that a perky couple came walking in the door hand-in-hand. When the front desk manager informed them that the regular teacher was not there, and that Darren Main would be filling in for him, they scoffed, and hurled a few insults at the front desk manager before storming out the door.

This couple clearly needed a yoga class, and thanks to their rude behavior, so did the girl working the desk. Now most people will not be quite so rude, but there is always a sense of disappointment on the part of students who come expecting one teacher only to find another teacher is there. That is the bad news.

The good news is that yoga students will often get in a rut with one or two teachers, and won't even consider working with teachers who are new to them. When they show up and a sub is filling in, their initial reaction may be one of disappointment, but if you do your job well, you may just open their minds up to new expressions of their practice, including, perhaps, taking some of your other classes.

In order to get the most from subbing, I recommend a few things.

1. Welcome feedback and comments. If someone likes your class, invite them to fill out a comment card for the management.

2. Have printed schedules. People will forget you before they get to the car if you don't put something in their hands.

3. Put your mailing list out so interested people can give you their contact info.

IMPORTANT: Subbing is NOT about stealing another teacher's students. It is unethical to do this, and it is counterproductive from a marketing standpoint. Most of the people in that room will be there because they really like the regular teacher. If you compliment that teacher, and tell the students what an honor it was to teach for him/her, they will respect you and be much more likely to expand their weekly practice to include both of you. Teaching yoga should never be a competition between teachers.

Network with Other Professionals

Free

Not a day goes by when a student doesn't ask me for a referral to a doctor, chiropractor, physical therapist, psychologist, or some other type of professional. Having a list of professionals you know are both talented and ethical is essential.

For many years, yoga teachers and other professionals seemed to be at odds. Sadly it was common to hear yoga teachers trash western doctors and other professionals. This, of course, did not go over well in the medical community, and they in turn did not view our profession as legitimate. Thankfully that has changed. As more and more yoga teachers have stopped the self-defeating practice of talking badly about other professions, those professionals have given yoga another look, and they tend to like what they see. Many often counsel their clients to practice yoga on a regular basis.

One should never refer a student unless there is a genuine need, but when a need exists, be sure to give the student a referral. This is simultaneously good for the student, and it's great marketing. Who do you think that doctor will think of next time one of her patients is in need of some yoga? Is it likely that the psychotherapist you refer to will encourage his clients to take your yoga classes when he knows you value his work!

Building a strong network of professionals to whom you can refer is a great way to support your existing students and garner new ones. Healing is often more effective with a multi-dimensional approach.

Network with Other Teachers

Free

Several months ago, a woman began taking my restorative class following a recent hysterectomy. Although her surgeon had cleared her to do yoga, she was still in a great deal of discomfort from the resulting scar tissue. Within a few weeks the soothing restorative yoga poses had significantly reduced her discomfort, but the months of recovery had prevented her from exercise. As a result she had gained nearly thirty pounds.

While her recovery was progressing nicely, she was still not ready for my more active vinyasa class, so I suggested she take a gentle hatha class with another teacher at Yoga Tree. I explained to her that this gentle class would be more active than my restorative class, but still considerably more mellow than my hatha flow class, and it would be a good way for her to ease into a more active practice.

She took my advice and did start taking a gentle class. A week later, Lauren Slater [www.laurenslateryoga.com], the teacher to whom I had referred her thanked me for the referral. But something else started to happen as well. I started seeing new students show up in my class who had been referred by Lauren.

When we refer to other teachers who offer classes that might be more appropriate for a given student, we create a culture in which everyone wins. The student wins because they are getting the instruction that is most appropriate for their needs. Your fellow yoga teachers win because they benefit from the word-of-mouth marketing and you win because in doing what is right for your students, you are creating a professional culture in which other teachers stop seeing you as competition and start seeing you as a colleague.

We have nothing to fear in referring our students to other teachers and styles of yoga, but we have everything to gain. I have seen my willingness to send students to other teachers result, not in a loss of students in my class, but rather in a rich and fertile community in which other teachers refer to me more freely, and my students feel that I'm looking out for their best interests.

Join Professional Organizations

Low Cost

There are many local, national, and even international professional organizations where you can share ideas, find other professionals to whom you can refer, and hopefully learn a few tips and tricks for effective business skills and marketing.

Some organizations, such as The Chamber of Commerce are general in nature, while other groups are for more specific types of professionals. There are groups for professional women, ethnic minorities, lesbians and gay men, and many more. These groups may or may not be specific to yoga, but remember, some of your best referrals will come from other professionals in the broader community.

A few years ago a woman took my class who had been referred to me by her divorce attorney. Yoga teachers and divorce attorneys seemingly have little in common, but I had met the divorce attorney at a professional mixer, and she thought that my yoga class would help her client manage the considerable stress of going through a particularly messy divorce.

Here are a few things you can do to maximize the benefits:

◊ Attend meetings and mixers regularly.

◊ Contribute articles or essays to the group's newsletter.

◊ Offer a merchant discount or a free class to members.

◊ Link to their website.

◊ List your membership with professional organizations on your resume.

◊ Offer to teach a class or workshop for the members.

Endorsements

Free

There is something powerful about being endorsed by someone who has taken your class and had a life-changing experience as a result. How many times have you gone to a restaurant, seen a movie, or checked out a massage therapist because a friend told you about their experience? The same is obviously true for yoga teachers.

Posting endorsements on your website and in other promotional material is an easy way to inspire people to take your class. There are three types of endorsements to seek out. Each carries with it slightly different benefits.

Student Endorsements

There is perhaps nothing more persuasive than the testimony of a satisfied student. Any nice things you say about yourself can easily come across as self-serving and egotistical, but a student singing your praises will speak volumes, as they have nothing to gain. They are speaking about their experience.

The next time a student emails you or approaches you after class to compliment you, ask them if they would be willing to write a few sentences endorsing your class. It's important not to be pushy, but in most cases you won't need to be. In fact, most students are honored to do it. You can then take that endorsement and post it to your website. Be sure to include their name and profession, as that will make them seem more real, and professional titles will lend more credibility to their words.

Sample:

My doctors recommended I take yoga for my tight lower back. I was skeptical about it helping, but after my first class with Jennifer Jones, I felt instant relief from my discomfort. The pain has steadily decreased ever since, and my regular visits to her class keep me pain free. Jennifer's gentleness and knowledge helped me to regain my mobility.

—John Smith, Accountant, Chicago, IL.,

Senior Teacher Endorsements

When my second book, *Yoga and the Path of the Urban Mystic*, was first released, I was relatively unknown outside San Francisco. So I decided to write to a number of well-known teachers whom I held in high regard to ask them if I could send them a copy of the manuscript for review. Some didn't bother to write back; others wrote back and said they didn't have the time, but a surprising number of very well-known teachers did take the time to read the manuscript and offered stellar endorsements.

I can't tell you how many times studios in cities around the world have hired me to teach workshops for them based on those endorsements alone. To this day I get emails from readers who have enjoyed the book, but only picked it up initially because John Friend [www.anusara.com], Judith Hanson Lasater [www.judithlasater.com], or Sharon Gannon [www. jivamuktiyoga.com] had endorsed it.

If you have a relationship with a senior yoga teacher, whether they are internationally known, or a local teacher who is well regarded in your area, ask them if they would be willing to write a blurb for you to post on your website. Getting up the nerve to ask can be difficult, and you may get some rejections, but more often than not, I have found that most teachers are honored by the request and are thrilled to support newer teachers.

The following is an endorsement that I wrote for one of the teachers who went through the teacher training I run at Yoga Tree.

> *Michael Alexander [www.alexanderyoga.com] is a skilled yoga teacher and a powerful healer. He uses both his knowledge of yoga and his own healing journey to inspire anyone lucky enough to practice with him.*

—*Darren Main, author of* Yoga and the Path of the Urban Mystic

Other Professional Endorsements

"Nine out of ten doctors recommend . . ." or so begins almost every commercial for over-the-counter pain relievers. How many times have you seen a poster for a new drug with a photo of a handsome doctor in a white lab coat and stethoscope, with his arms folded across his broad chest? I'm not sure if they hand-select the doctors or pay them to recommend their drug, or even if the models are actual doctors, but one thing I do know is that people trust doctors and other professionals. Even the suggestion that a doctor endorses a product gives it credibility.

Most professionals carry clout with the population at large, and sporting a professional endorsement on your website is a fantastic way to inspire the confidence of students who may not know you. Like all other endorsements, it is important that you ask professionals in a respectful manner, but if you have a relevant professional such as a chiropractor, psychotherapist, clergy member, or doctor, who has seen the value of yoga generally, and your class in particular, ask if they would be willing to write a short blurb. In exchange you can always link to their website.

Sample:

> *Having treated thousands of cancer patients over the years, I have seen few things ease the side effects of chemotherapy and radiation like Jennifer Smith's restorative yoga class. With her gentle guidance my patients are able to breathe and relax, allowing them to tolerate treatments with greater ease and access the body's inherent ability to heal.*

—*John Smith, M.D., Oncologist, Detroit General Hospital*

Religious and Community Groups

Free

Some religious groups are opposed to yoga, believing it conflicts with their church doctrines, but many see yoga as a great complement to what they are offering. Here in San Francisco, I teach a weekly class inside the world famous Grace Cathedral on the large marble labyrinth that is inlaid on the floor. The church is thrilled to have me there, as it helps their congregation to explore the "body temple" referred to by Saint Paul in the Bible [1Corinthians 6:19-20] and brings new people, who are not regular church-goers, into the church. For me, it is really fun to teach in such a majestic space, and people who might otherwise be afraid of yoga feel affirmed by the fact that the church embraces it.

Working with churches and synagogues is a great way to reach out to people who might not otherwise consider yoga, and most religious groups have built-in marketing with church bulletins, websites, and announcements.

In addition, if you belong to a particular religion, you can offer to hold a fundraiser class or workshop for them, or contribute an article or essay about yoga for their newsletter. All this gets your name out there and invites a very targeted group of people to explore yoga in a way that is non-threatening to their faith.

Joint Workshops

Earn You Money

Workshops are a great way to take your students to a deeper level of practice, but they can be a lot of work in terms of planning, marketing, and holding the space needed for a successful experience. Sometimes, working with another teacher is a great way to share that burden and lend credibility to the workshop as well

I used to teach a workshop at a local gym with one of the personal trainers, called, "Yoga & Weight Training." By working with him, we increased our outreach, the appeal of the workshop, and turned a lot of folks on to yoga who had never considered the practice as a complement to their weight training. Since I had a personal trainer working with me, most people felt that it wasn't just a pitch to get them to let go of the weights, but rather the chance to integrate the two forms of exercise. Consequently, the workshops were consistently sold out. Better still, many of the people who attended the workshop went on to become my regular students.

If you feel a passion for working with a certain issue, find another yoga teacher or professional who can offer a joint workshop with you. If you want to work with depression, maybe you could find a psychologist to share the workshop. If you want to work with children, offer a workshop with a schoolteacher. Maybe you want to teach a workshop on core strength—you could join forces with a local Pilates teacher. The possibilities are endless.

Live Music

Free/low cost

As I previously mentioned, I teach a weekly class in San Francisco's Grace Cathedral. The beautiful gothic church is a spectacular place to practice yoga amidst the stained glass windows, lofty ceilings, and beautiful statues.

Shortly after I started the class I contacted my friend Sam Jackson [www. vibrantstillness.com], whose renowned CD, *Dropping into Stillness*, is a staple in many yoga classes. Sam's singing crystal bowls are deeply moving and inspire a deep state of meditation. He was excited to join me once a month playing live music.

The class has grown from about twenty people per week to over two hundred students. In addition to Sam, I have since asked a number of well-known local and traveling musicians to join me, including Christopher Love [www. lovechristopher.com], Timothy Das [www.harmonicdreams.com], Mirabai [www.mirabaiandfriends.com], Jonathan Wolf [www.dragonflutesrising. com], and Kendra Faye. The thrill of practicing yoga set to live music in such a sacred space is attracting people from all walks of life.

Many local musicians are looking for venues where they can introduce people to their music, and this is especially true of musicians who play World music, New Age music, or chant, as radio stations are generally unwilling to play their music.

Be sure to limit the invitations to musicians who play music appropriate to your class and teaching style. This is a great win for your students, for the musicians, and for yourself!

Continue Your Education

Low Cost

Aside from being an important part of growing as a professional, continuing your education is a great way to network with other teachers, to share marketing ideas, and to gain valuable insights as to how you can grow your business.

If you are doing something unique, be sure to have your elevator pitch ready. That way, when other teachers ask you about that unique class you are teaching for troubled youth, cancer patients, or women suffering from lupus, you will have a ready answer, and they will be able to refer students your way.

Continuing education keeps your teaching fresh and exciting, and sharing ideas with other yoga teachers helps you. We don't need to reinvent the wheel. If another teacher has lead a retreat or worked at a particular gym, they will probably have some valuable advice for you.

Yoga Conferences

Expensive

Every year there are numerous yoga conferences in a variety of cities around the world. These conferences give you the opportunity both to continue your education and to network with the larger community of teachers beyond your local region.

While attending these conferences can be expensive, they easily pay for themselves in the connections you can make, as well as the ways in which they can inspire you as a teacher. It's not uncommon for the teachers in an area to get burdened with stale ideas. By stepping out and experiencing teachers to whom you don't regularly have access, you will often bring fresh ideas, techniques, and inspiration back home to your classes. Your students will feel this injection of fresh energy and will in turn become more excited about your classes.

Yoga Journal offers a number of conferences each year which bring together some of the biggest names in yoga. While *Yoga Journal* is not the only group offering conferences, they are certainly the largest [www.yogajournal.com/conferences].

Pro Bono Work

Free

If you feel passionately about helping a particular group of people who might not be able to afford yoga, you will love doing pro bono work. We often get so focused on making yoga a business that we can lose passion for what we are doing. When you volunteer your time, you get so much in return. Whether you teach at a jail or a drug rehab facility, a battered women's shelter, or even at your child's school, you will find that you can deepen your teaching and create a much more colorful resume at the same time.

I can't put my finger on why doing pro bono work is such an effective marketing tool, but I can tell you that, without exception, doing volunteer work has always produced more for me than I could ever give out. The

Wiccan religion has a doctrine known as the "three-fold law," in which they believe that any energy you put out will come back to you three times stronger. If you put out negative, harmful energy, you will receive it back three times stronger. If, however, you are generous with your kindness and compassion, the world returns that positive energy three times over.

In addition to the good karma, many media outlets are looking for feel-good stories to cover. The fact that you teach a yoga class at the local YMCA is not really newsworthy. The fact that you are volunteering at a drug rehab facility is far more likely to catch the eye of a reporter—especially if you send out a press release calling their attention to the class.

Nonprofit Fundraising

Free

Nonprofit groups are almost always struggling. They need support and will welcome most offers to help out. What's more, they will promote your name and your classes heavily, as their ability to raise money from your work is tied to turnout. Similar to pro bono work, media outlets will often sit up and take notice.

There are a number of ways you can support your favorite nonprofit organizations:

◊ Offer free classes to be raffled.

◊ Teach a class or workshop, and give the money you raise to their organization.

◊ Teach classes for fundraising events such as walkathons, marathons, or bicycle riding to raise money.

Print Marketing
Quality Design

Moderate Cost

Compare the fast food hamburger and fries you get at the drive through window to the images you see on their advertising. The ad will likely sport crisp lettuce, a bright red tomato, and fries that are cooked to a perfect golden crisp. The real life meal will offer you a soggy bun, limp fries, and a tomato that tastes like cardboard. Yet, even though everyone knows the reality of fast food in both quality and health consequences, millions of people every day eat at greasy fast food chains.

Even though it is unethical to create images that are misleading, many fast food chains do. The good news is, yoga teachers don't need to do that. To have pleasing, well-designed print marketing, which conveys the essence of what you are offering is not unethical in the least. In fact, it is really being honest about what you offer.

A surprising number of yoga teachers try to design flyers, postcards, and the like on the cheap, and the result is tacky and unattractive. Worse still, poorly designed marketing material can actually drive students away. The next time you are at a local café, look at the flyers hanging on their community board. Notice the ones that catch your eye and evoke an emotional response. Notice also the ones that are fit for little more than lining the bottom of a bird cage.

If you don't have design skills, invest in a professional who can help! If you do want to design on your own, keep the following tips in mind.

Less is More

If you try to cram too much text into a flyer, people won't read it. A certain amount of white space is necessary. Keep it short and sweet, and provide people with a way to get more information once you whet their appetite.

Easy on the Color

Flyers that look like a child ate a box of crayons and then vomited onto the page are tacky. Unless you are marketing to Rainbow Brite, choose two or three colors at most. The colors should catch the eye without being so loud that they distract from the serenity that yoga offers.

Easy on the Fonts

Just because your computer has hundreds of fonts to choose from doesn't mean you should use all of them on a single page. Choose one or two fonts and make sure they are easy to read.

Centering is for the Meditation Cushion

Centering everything on your flyer is not recommended and difficult for the eye to follow. Small bite size blocks of text are generally best.

Photos should inspire—not terrify

How many times have you seen a poster in which the yoga teacher is featured doing some crazy pose that looks impossible to obtain and unpleasant to execute. Your flyers are not supposed to stroke your ego; they are supposed to inspire people to take your class or workshop. Tasteful, elegant, and attainable poses are far more attractive. Photos of students having a good time—even smiling—will have the same effect.

One of the biggest mistakes new yoga teachers make on their flyers, as well as on their websites, is that they use photos of themselves in very difficult poses. This fails on several fronts. First, the class is not about you; it is about your students. Therefore, a photo should convey to potential students what they can expect to learn and how you can help them learn it.

Second, while a photo of you standing on one hand may be impressive, you need to remember that you are not advertising a circus act. While potential students may look at that photo with awe, they may also decide that your class is not for them. It is for this reason that you should choose poses that are elegant, yet attainable for the students you are trying to reach.

For example, let's say you want to build a flyer for a senior citizen's yoga class that you are going to be offering at a local community center. Having a photo of you standing on your head is going to scare off the people you are trying to reach. Rather than a photo of you, find a senior to model for you, and have them do a pose that looks fun and attainable. Make sure they are smiling or have a look of peace. If you must be in the photo, have it be as a teacher gently assisting the model. In this way, the seniors who see the photo will feel welcome and will know something about what they can expect from the class.

By using a combination of images, text, colors, and fonts, your flyers should answer one question for the person who picks it up. "What's in it for me?" If you produce a flyer that's a confusing jumble of text and color, adorned with photos of you doing unappealing yoga poses, you will not answer that basic question.

Business Cards

Low Cost

Not a day goes by when someone doesn't ask me what I do for a living. It seems to be a national conversation piece that rivals talking about the weather. For the most part people don't really care about the answer—they simply want to fill the empty spaces with meaningless conversation.

The bad news is none of us can escape this small talk. The good news is you have a job that is unique and interesting to a fairly large segment of the population. Thus, when I tell people that I teach yoga they naturally want to know more. I generally get peppered with questions such as:

"What kind of yoga do you teach?"

"Would yoga be good for my injury or illness?"

"Can you put your foot behind your head?"

If yoga is appropriate for them, which in most cases it is, I hand them a business card and write on the back, "one free class." Everyone likes getting free stuff, and I feel quite confident that if they take a class, they will keep coming back. There is no need to give a high-powered sales pitch. The yoga will sell itself, but giving them your business card may be just the nudge they need to try yoga.

Like flyers, it is important that your cards are professionally designed and inspire confidence in you as a teacher. In addition, when you network with other professionals, such as doctors and psychotherapists, the design of your card is going to go a long way in their willingness to hand them out to their clients.

Many years ago, my Uncle Peter began selling real estate. His office was competitive, and everyone was printing up flashy business cards sporting their educational letters. Since Peter didn't have a PhD or any degree that would bolster his image, he put the letters RBM.

In most cases, people would just assume that RBM was some sort of impressive credential and, not wanting to appear uninformed about what it stood for, they would not ask. Occasionally a curious person would ask what RBM stood for and Peter would have a great laugh with them when he explained that it stood for Rapidly Becoming a Millionaire. This put people at ease with Peter, and he went on to make a considerable amount of money selling commercial real estate. Much of Peter's success was due to his willingness to be himself, just as he represented on his business cards.

Schedules

Low Cost

Naturally you should post your schedule to your website, but in today's fast-paced world, many people forget all about you and your website minutes after you chat with them. Therefore, it's important to put something in their hand when they request more information about your classes.

When I first moved to San Francisco, my classes were rather small, since no one knew me yet. As a result, I would regularly sub for more established teachers. Often, students would like my class and ask about my regular classes. Rather than simply handing them a card that would likely get lost in the bottom of their bag, I handed them a printed copy of my schedule. This way they could start planning to attend one of my classes the moment they saw my schedule.

Like your other printed material, your schedule should be tastefully designed and should include the times, locations, and levels of each class. It is also wise to put your website and other contact information on the schedule, and when appropriate, you can write "one free class" on the schedule to give them an added incentive to attend.

Flyers & Postcards

Moderate Cost

Many cafés, health food stores, and community centers have public boards on which you can leave flyers and postcards. This is a low cost way to market yourself, but there are a few things to remember.

◊ Always ask before posting. Many establishments require the approval of the management before posting flyers. If you post without asking there is a good chance your flyer will be discarded and you will alienate a potential marketing resource.

◊ Find out when various establishments clear their boards. Many will have a monthly day on which they toss everything into the recycling bin. If you can post just after they clear the board, you will get prime real estate, and your flyer will have a much longer shelf life.

◊ Have your flyers and postcards professionally designed. Take a visit to your local café and notice the flyers hanging on the wall. Which ones catch your eye? Which flyers blend in and become paper white noise? When I stopped trying to save money by designing my own print material, I noticed a precipitous increase in the return on my investment.

◊ Have your flyers and postcards professionally printed on glossy, colored paper. This will cost more, but will dramatically increase their effectiveness.

Coupon Books

Moderate to Expensive Cost

Most areas have coupon books or flyers that get mailed out or stuffed into newspapers. The nice thing about coupon books is that you are sharing the marketing expenses with other businesses, and you are reaching a very broad audience. You will want to make sure, however, that you are the only yoga teacher advertising in a given book. By giving away a free class you will likely get a lot of new students, and because they will need to bring the coupon when they come to class, you will have a clear indication of just how well that coupon book worked. If there is more than one teacher offering classes, the chances that people will drift from teacher to teacher are greatly increased.

Print Ads

Expensive

Running an ad in a newspaper or magazine is a great way to get the word out about your classes, but it doesn't come cheap. What's more, you may not see results in the short term, as research suggests that a person needs to see an advertisement at least six times, and as many as twelve, before they take the leap and buy a product or service. This means that you will probably need to run an ad for a number of consecutive issues before you see results.

Given the pricey nature of print advertisements, many yoga teachers choose to forego this option. There are, however, certain circumstances in which running an ad may be well worth the investment. Generally, this is the case when you are offering something that is very unique.

Several years ago, I was offering a yoga class for people with HIV. I took out a small ad in the local gay paper and requested they place the advertisement next to articles on HIV. The response was quite impressive and the new students the ad brought in easily paid for the steep price.

Tip: If you offer a discount or a free class when they mention the advertisement, you will often see a greater return on your investment. In addition, it will help you to gauge the effectiveness of the ad.

Web-Based Marketing

The World Wide Web has given us many things—cute videos of animals and children, instant access to news, and the ability to communicate with people all over the world.

Readers of a certain age will remember a thing called the Yellow Pages. Ask yourself this: "When was the last time I opened the big yellow book?" People now go to Google for their answers. If you don't have a web presence very few people will be able to find you. Having a web presence is fairly easy and very inexpensive, but some personal reflection and mindfulness is essential. Remember, the content you put on the internet will be your introduction to students. If your web presence is sloppy and not well planned, you can actually do more harm than good.

Website

Low Cost

There is nothing more important in today's marketing world than having your own website. If you do nothing else, create a personal website! It is one of the cheapest and most effective ways to communicate with your current students, and introduce yourself to new ones.

In the next chapter I will be covering some basic design principles and how to get started. For now, suffice it to say that your website should be clean, easy to navigate, and provide information about you, your teaching style, your schedule, and any other information that might inspire people to take your classes and workshops.

Tip: All roads lead to your website. Your website should be everywhere—on your business cards and flyers, on your Facebook page, and on your teacher bio page at the studios where you teach. You should mention it if you are on TV or radio, and you should always remember that your website represents you! It could be the deciding factor in whether or not a potential student will make the leap and take your class! Like the clothes you wear, your hair style, and other accents, your website will help potential students define you for better or worse, so put some thought into the presence you want to create and the types of students with which you want to work.

Search Engines

Free

Search engines like Google have changed the way we find information. If you want potential students to find you, you will need to understand how search engines like Google function. While each search engine is a bit different under the hood, there are a number of things you can do to get noticed and listed.

If you simply post something to the internet, search engines will eventually find you. They use complex programs called 'crawlers' or 'spiders' that spend every second of every day surfing the internet and cataloging what they find. If for example, you put the word 'yoga' on your website and someone types in the word 'yoga,' your site will be listed once a crawler has visited your site.

Of course there are a few problems with this. First, you don't necessarily want to wait for Yahoo, Google, and Ask.com to stumble across your site. It could take months before they find you. Second, even after they do find and index your site, there is nothing saying you will turn up at the top of the list of search results. In fact, you may be so far down the list that no one will ever find you. So let's take a look at how to improve your odds.

The fastest way to get a search engine to find your website is to invite their crawler to visit you. On every search engine's page—usually hidden near the bottom in very small text, is a link that says something like "submit URL" or "submit website." If you click on that link you will be guided through a submission process. Even doing this, it may take time before a crawler visits your site, but generally speaking, it will cut your wait time.

Since every search engine has its own submission page, you will need to invest some time to make sure you get listed in as many engines as possible. There are services out there, which, for a fee, will submit your site to multiple engines for you. These services are usually a waste of money and should normally be avoided.

Before you submit your site, however, be sure you have key words embedded in your site. This can be done in two basic ways. First, the text of your site should be picked up quickly. That said, graphics that contain text would not be readable to the crawlers. For example, if you have a menu or a title bar in jpeg or gif format, any text in those graphics will not help you.

A second way to have your site indexed properly is through the use of metta tags. These tags are invisible to the casual viewer, but crawlers will read them easily. Basically, metta tags are lists of key words buried in the code of your site.

My website, for example, might include the following tags: darren, main, San Francisco, yoga, meditation, pranayama, breathwork, urban mystic, inner tranquility, yogi entrepreneur, retreats, and so on.

Your webmaster can help you with this, but if you have a list of key words separated by commas, it will help your webmaster greatly.

Getting to the Top of the Heap

In a moment, I will be discussing Ad Words—which is a way to pay to get your website to come up on top. There are techniques to increase your site showing on various search engines called, Search Engine Optimization (SEO). In fact, there are companies that specialize in SEO work and charge a hefty sum for their services. While each engine has its own algorithm for determining how important a website is, most of them involve the hyperlinks associated with your site. Sites that have a lot of links on them generally have a better showing on search engines, as do sites that a lot of other sites link to.

It is for this reason that you should link to as many relevant sites as possible, and encourage others to link to your site as well. The more students, friends, family, and any other yoga-related websites who link to your site, the higher you will show up in search engine results.

Three Tips for Improving Search Results

◊ Resource Page- Link to all relevant sites.

◊ Blog- The more you blog, the more noteworthy your site will be to search engines. Always include useful links in your blog entries.

◊ Write articles and submit them to as many blogs as possible. You can even use an article submission service to syndicate your articles. Always include a link to your site at the end of the piece.

The next chapter will help you map out your website and learn some web design basics so you can work with your web designer to create an attractive and informative site, as well as one that will be easy for search engines to catalog.

Tip: Google offers a free Key Word Research Tool, which can help you determine which key words are best for your site [https://adwords.google.com/select/KeywordToolExternal].

Email List

Moderate Cost

Your ability to communicate with your students is perhaps the most important thing you can develop. In years past this meant shelling out money for postage and printing. It also meant a lot of dead trees. With email, these costs are greatly reduced. Understanding how email works is important, however.

The Spam Free Zone

Email is so cheap that less than reputable people have decided to spam— that is, send unsolicited emails to as many people as possible. They know that most people will simply delete the garbage they send, but when they lard up the net with millions of messages per day, they are aware that even if a small percentage of the people they spam will fall for their ploy, they will cash in big time.

Internet service providers and email clients, like Apple Mail and Microsoft Outlook, have tried to address this by creating junk mail filters that block servers to those who send out unsolicited emails to large groups of people. The good news is that this helps reduce the amount of junk email you have to wade through. The bad news is that these filters can't always tell the difference between what is solicited (people who have requested to be on your mailing list) and what is unsolicited (people sending rubbish to every email address they can find).

If you want to email a group of students, your message will likely be blocked if you don't do it the right way. Simply copying a list of addresses into a message is likely to land your email newsletter in the junk mail folder, but there are services out there that can help.

My personal favorite is iContact, but it is certainly not the only reputable company. Services like iContact have a relationship with most internet service providers. In exchange for emails sent through their service skirting past filters, these companies agree to police their members. If you send unsolicited spam emails they will promptly drop you.

In addition to helping you separate your email blasts from those who are selling cheap Viagra and mail order brides, they provide valuable tracking services and allow you to send HTML emails embedded with links, graphics, and photos. Many even provide templates to help you design professional looking newsletters.

These services are not free, however. Generally they charge by the number of emails you send, and the number of email addresses in your list. Most new teachers will find that the cost is very reasonable, but it will go up over time as your email list continues to grow.

White Noise

The biggest mistake made by a number of teachers is in the number of emails they send. When your emails become a burden to your students they will simply hit delete without bothering to read them. Worse, they will unsubscribe from your list, or get so annoyed with you that they stop coming to your class. To send email blasts too frequently is like becoming annoying white noise in the inboxes of your students.

Rather than send out an email every week, send out a monthly newsletter, and make sure there is something of interest to your students beyond a sales pitch for your classes. Perhaps you could include a short informative article or a pose of the month. In other words, give your students a reason to open your emails rather than deleting them.

Yoga Teacher Directories

Moderate Cost/Low cost

There are a number of teacher directories for all students to search, based on location and style. Some are focused on a particular style. For example, Judith Hanson Lasater hosts a directory for restorative yoga teachers [www.dragonflutesrising.com] who have completed her training. Others are more general and list a number of teachers and styles.

Ad Words

Low to Moderate Cost

Facebook, Google, and other search engines and social networking sites offer what are commonly called ad words. Basically, you bid on search terms and key words, and if your bid is the highest, a link or ad will be displayed. In the case of Google, the ad will be listed at the top of the search results or on the sidebar. In the case of Facebook, the ad will be listed on various pages you visit. The more money you bid, the more likely your ad is to get prominent placement.

TIPS: *Choose key words that will uniquely apply to you.* For example, I might choose "restorative, yoga, San Francisco." You want to be specific, but not so specific that your listing never pops up.

Pay by View: When you choose pay by view, you are paying for someone to see your listing. This doesn't mean they click on it to be taken to your site. It simply means they see it. The benefit is that you generally pay less per view. The bad news is that many web ads have become like white noise, so your ad may get tuned out.

Pay per Click: When you opt to pay per click, you are only paying for people who actually click through to your website. This doesn't guarantee you will have a new student, but at least they took the time to check out your site. The down side is this mode usually costs a bit more.

Know your budget: Most ad word programs allow you to set a budget limit per day. The amount is up to you, but if you want a lot of eyes on your ad, then you will want to set the budget limit as high as you can afford.

Blogging

Free

In the age of blogging many people fancy themselves a journalist and a poet. Most blogs are self-indulgent, but if done right, you can develop a following that will bring readers to your site over and over again. It's important to remember that unique, relevant content is what brings people back.

Maybe you have a yoga pose of the week in which you describe the pose, its benefits, precautions, and modifications. Or maybe you will post relevant videos from YouTube. (They can even be your own.) You can write essays or share inspiring stories about students (with their permission of course). The richer the content, the better!

There are several ways to set up a blog. The easiest is to set up a free account with a service like Google or Word Press. In addition, there is software that can be used to help you tailor your blog to match your website. Word Press offers free software that can be installed on your website's server. While this is a bit technical to set up, once it is up and running, adding blog posts is quite simple. Your web designer can help you with the set-up process.

Podcasting

Free/Low cost

A few years back a San Diego based yoga teacher named Tim Jordan signed up for my annual yoga retreat in Joshua Tree [www.desertspiritretreat.com]. Since I had never met him, I was wondering how he found out about the retreat. He explained that he was an avid listener of my podcast, *Inquire Within* [www.inquirewithinpodcast.com].

It is very difficult to know specifically how effective my podcast is in increasing the attendance in my yoga classes, workshops, and retreats, but I'm sure it has been quite effective. People have come to my class from other countries when they pass through San Francisco, simply because they have heard my podcast.

A podcast is basically an internet radio or TV show that is syndicated to pod-catchers like iTunes, using a technology called "Really Simple Syndication" or RSS. Each time you post an episode, everyone who has subscribed to your podcast will automatically download that episode into their iPod or other MP3 player. In addition, gadgets like TIVO, XBOX, and even some DVD players can download the podcasts to which a person subscribes.

The nice thing about podcasts is that they can be targeted. For example, my podcast features interviews with authors, healers, teachers, and musicians in the yoga and spiritual communities. Unlike NPR, which reaches many more people, my podcast is syndicated to those people who have a passion for all things having to do with yoga. If you decide to produce your own podcast, you will want to really think about who will be listening. If, for example, you are a prenatal teacher, you might want to interview people who are birthing experts, such as midwives, OBGYNs, authors of books about pregnancy, and even women who had a positive experience with pregnancy and birthing because of yoga.

If the technical side of podcasting is overwhelming, fear not. There are resources to make the experience pain free even if you are a technophobe. Here are a few resources to get you started:

Liberated Syndication
[www.libsyn.com]

For a surprisingly small fee, this website will host your podcast and syndicate it to iTunes and many other pod catchers. You don't even need to know how to spell RSS, and you can set the template for your podcast page to match your website. Posting new episodes is as easy as point and click.

Podcast Solutions: The Complete Guide to Podcasting
by Michael Geoghegan and Dan Klass

This book is the podcaster's bible. It will guide you through every step of the process, from choosing the right microphone, to software and promotion. It is available as a paperback or eBook.

Behringer PodcaStudio

If you are overwhelmed with which microphone and sound board to choose, this package by Behringer is your dream come true. Set-up is effortless, and it has everything you need to get started.

Software

When you record your podcast, you will need to edit it. This may sound hard, but with the right software, it is quite easy. Here are a few low cost options for you to consider:

Audacity (OS X, Windows)- This open source software is free, so you can't beat the price. It is not as polished or intuitive as some of the applications you pay for, but it is a great place to start [www.audacity.sourceforge.net].

Wiretap Studio (OS X)- If you are going to be recording phone/Skype interviews, this is your best option. It allows you to edit each track separately so you can clean up and adjust the volume of the person you are interviewing. It can be used as a stand-alone piece of software or in conjunction with other applications [www.ambrosiasw.com].

GarageBand (OS X)- This is perhaps the easiest audio editing software for the Mac, and it comes free with every new computer. It makes recording, editing, and publishing easy. You can even compose music, sound effects, and put filters on your voice to make the episode sound very professional [www.apple.com].

Facebook

Free

I knew Facebook was big when my mother posted her profile and started following my feeds. Facebook and other social networking sites allow you to do a number of things at no cost. First, it lets your students and potential students get to know you better. They can see what kinds of movies you like, what kinds of books you read, and they can see photos of you, both as a teacher and a 'real person.' It also enables you to announce new classes, workshops, and events. Finally, it is a great way to link back to your own website.

Warning: Young people today have an expression: T.M.I (too much information). While I'm a big fan of social networking sites and posting regular, honest information about yourself, your interests, and the news and events from your life, there is such a thing as being too open. It is not necessarily in your best professional interest for your students to know about the argument you had with your spouse, or the fact that you think the owner of your yoga studio is a jerk. There are no hard lines about what to post and what not to post, but if you have any doubt about posting something personal, you probably shouldn't be posting it!

Tip: Be a good Facebook citizen. It's okay to post the occasional workshop announcement on your wall, but try to mix it up with other fun and informative posts. People who are always selling something lose credibility in the social networking community. Consider the following recent posts to my wall:

Darren is packing for his retreat to India.

Darren is laughing at a funny video on YouTube.

Darren has a new yoga class for strengthening the immune system.

Darren just had an amazing lunch at the Samovar Tea Lounge.

As you can see, only one of them is an overt advertisement for my teaching, but in spite of that, I have conveyed a number of details. People know I'm leading a retreat to India, that I like eating at a certain restaurant, and that I enjoy funny YouTube videos as much as the next guy.

In the case of the funny video, I posted it to my blog. In this way followers of my post who want a good laugh can do it at my website, where they will hopefully spend some time surfing around the rest of the site.

Twitter

Free

Micro-blogging with services like twitter can be fun or annoying, depending on your perspective. Like Facebook, be sure to consider carefully what you post. If you are taking your dog to the vet to get checked for worms, your students probably don't need to know that. Short, little blasts of wisdom, announcements about upcoming classes and workshops, and some fun details about your life are all great uses for Twitter, as are links to yoga-related sites and news articles. You can even link your Twitter feed to your Facebook wall so you only have to post an announcement once.

Yelp!

Free/Expensive

Yelp and other consumer review sites are a great way to introduce new students to your class. Chances are that you will wind up on Yelp whether you like it or not, since anyone can post a Yelp review. What you can do is make sure that your presence on Yelp is pleasing and informative, and you can link to it from your website.

There is a down side to Yelp, however. Not everyone is going to like you, and some people will want to tell the world just what a bad teacher you are. Several years ago, a woman named Lauren posted the following review about me:

> *Darren Main was nothing more than a disappointment. He is arrogant, rigid, and patronizing. He runs the Yoga Tree Teacher Training with a condescending air and general indifference to the needs of the trainees.*
>
> *Hot stones can't save his Restorative Yoga classes at Yoga Tree Stanyan. Thank God for his dedicated and helpful assistants otherwise that class would have been a total waste of $17.*
>
> *The Hatha Flow All Levels at Yoga Tree Stanyan is no better. The space is jam packed with little room to move. I understand what 'flow' means, but shouldn't you be able to take at least half a breath every third pose? He does not give due attention to newcomers either. It's every yogi and yogini for themselves.*

Unfortunately for me, she never discussed her feelings with me before posting this blistering rebuke, and that review will live on Yelp for the rest of time. The good news is that her negative review is mixed in with a sea of other very positive reviews. The bad news is that it is out on the web for the whole world to see, and there is nothing I can do about it.

Your first public critique will likely sting. I know teachers who have cried themselves to sleep over bad reviews. When you put yourself out there in the public eye, some people will love you; others will hate you. It may not be fair, but it is a reality.

The internet has given people permission to write hurtful things with little or no consequences to temper their tirades. Yelp is a magnet for people like this. Unfortunately, there is nothing we can do about it. If you own a business, people will review it, and some of them will say unflattering things. The best we can do is invite our loyal students to write reviews as well, so that the negative comments are drowned out in good reviews. On the whole, Yelp and sites like it are a huge perk for businesses small and large. You simply need to have faith that if you provide a quality product at a fair price, most people will sing your praises.

Yelp is a free service for the most part, but if you want your Yelp page to come up at the top of searches, you can pay them to have your listing bumped to the top. This generally gets you more reviews and puts your name and website in front of a lot more eyeballs than taking the free option. Of course, you can always start with the free option, and then contact their sales office to upgrade at any time.

Linkedin

Free

Linkedin is a great site that allows you to connect with other professionals. In many ways it resembles Facebook, but with a decided bent toward networking. Not a day goes by when a doctor, chiropractor, or psychotherapist doesn't refer a student to my class. In the past, we needed to spend hours pounding the pavement to talk to other professionals. While Linkedin doesn't completely alleviate the need to network professionally the old fashioned way, it certainly makes it much easier.

HeartBeat.com

Free/low cost

HeartBeat.com provides one-stop shopping for busy yoga teachers. If Yelp and Twitter had a love child, it would be HeartBeat.com. It offers a lot of community based resources, event calendars, workshop registration services, and other useful tools for yoga teachers. HeartBeat.com will also tie together many other social networking sites such as Twitter and Facebook, so you can post to one spot and have the same post syndicated to a number of other venues with one click.

For example, suppose you are leading an *Intro to Meditation* workshop. Heartbeat.com can handle the registration of that workshop, and each time a student signs up for your workshop, an announcement can be automatically posted to their Facebook wall so others in their circle of friends can sign up too. Once they take your workshop and have an amazing time, they can go back to HeartBeat.com and write a great review that will help you promote your next meditation workshop. Best of all, this happens automatically.

This site offers a number of free services, as well as some advanced options for a small fee.

The Balance Market

Free/low cost

Thebalancemarket.com was created and designed by yoga teachers for yoga teachers. It's a resource hub geared toward practitioners looking for new ways to connect with their clients and find current industry news. The Balance Market team has designed easy-to-edit templates for business cards, newsletters, and much more, to help teachers maintain a professional look without breaking the bank. Check out the blog, which highlights industry-relevant products, inspirational teachers, and essential marketing tips so teachers can stay up-to-speed on what's happening in the field. Since they're committed to sustainable, earth-friendly practices, they love to feature products and people who strive for green business.

Yoga Journal Teacher Directory

Low Cost

Yoga Journal [www.yogajournal.com] is not just a magazine any more. They have a wonderful directory of yoga teachers and studios. For a very affordable price, you can list your name and even promote upcoming workshops and retreats. The will even list you in their mobile phone and tablet apps so people can find you on the go.

Book & Music Reviews

Free/pays you

Once you start teaching yoga you will start to feel like a miniature Oprah Winfrey. Students will continually ask you for book suggestions and music. With that in mind, why not turn that to your advantage. By reviewing your favorite books and music on Amazon, iTunes, and other related sites, your students will see your name out there. Remember, the more times someone sees your name, the more they will see you as a professional. Here are a few tips.

◊ Always include your full name, the fact that you are a yoga teacher, and whenever possible, your website.

◊ Copy and paste the review to a number of sites. If you're going to write a book review on Amazon, you might as well post it on Barnes & Noble's site as well.

◊ Write honest reviews, but avoid being a guttersnipe. Remember how it felt when you got that bad Yelp review, and avoid doing the same thing to someone else.

◊ Post your reviews to your blog. You can even set up an affiliate relationship with companies like Amazon, so that when someone buys something as a result of your website, they will give you a small commission for the referral.

Traditional Media
Database of Local Media

Free

In your local area, there are dozens, if not hundreds, of media outlets. Some of them are rather large, such as the evening news; others are smaller, such as local blogs covering what goes on in your area. Still others are medium-sized outlets, such as radio stations and weekly newspapers. In addition to mainstream media outlets that cover news and events generally, there are usually newsletters and websites devoted to sub-groups within your community. Each and every one of these outlets can be contacted with a press release each time you are doing something of note, and many will gladly cover your events if you know how to spin things.

In order to be most efficient, I suggest you start a database to easily sort through your media contacts—then add to it whenever you come across a media outlet in your area. The database need not be complicated. In fact, a simple excel spreadsheet will likely do the trick for most yoga teachers. Just be sure you collect as much information as you can, so that you can easily blast out press releases at a moment's notice.

Some things you might want to gather about media outlets in your database include:

◊ Name of Organization

◊ Contact Person Name

◊ Website of Organization

◊ Mailing Address

◊ Email

◊ Fax Number

◊ Submission Guidelines

◊ Type of Media (newspaper, radio, TV, etc.)

◊ Audience (general, religious, minority group, gay community, etc.)

◊ Coverage (local, state-wide, regional, national, international, etc.)

◊ Preferred method of contact (email, postal, phone, fax, etc.)

◊ Who Covered You in the Past? (Once you develop a relationship with an editor, producer, or reporter, getting coverage becomes easier.)

Tip: Whenever an organization covers you, be sure to send a handwritten thank you note. This will do more to get you repeat coverage than just about anything else. You can also include a free pass to one of your classes as an extra special thank you.

The Press Release

Free

A press release is basically an announcement inviting the media to cover your class, workshop, or event. It is one of the primary ways media outlets including TV, radio, podcasts, newspapers, blogs, and magazines become aware of newsworthy events.

The nice thing about a press release is that it's free to send one. The drawback is that because it's such a low cost way to promote, everybody and their dog sends them out. Really, though, you have nothing to lose and everything to gain. That said, if you want your press release to get more attention than the recycling bin, it's important that you observe a few rules.

◊ Reporters and producers are very, very busy. The press release should give them everything they need in a quick glance. If they want more information they can always contact you.

◊ In the clearest and most concise way possible it should contain the essentials of journalism: who, what, where, when and why.

◊ Always write the press release in the third person.

◊ If you have additional resources for them, let them know. This can include a free pass to your class, photos, and the link to the press section of your website, where they can get more information and download files, such as high resolution photos suitable for printing.

◊ If you're willing to give them an interview (which you should be!!) say so. If you have students with compelling stories who are willing to be interviewed, state that as well.

◊ Edit for grammar and spelling. Remember, most journalists studied English in college, and they can be very snooty when you butcher the language of their trade.

◊ Avoid all-caps, multi-colored, bright, flashy, difficult to read, and otherwise tacky fonts.

◊ Finally, write your release with the idea that it is not a sales pitch for a used car. A good reporter can sniff out a good story. The press release is there to inspire them to think about the story and to envision that story being told by them.

Elements of a Press Release

◊ Logo/Photo

◊ Contact Information

◊ Title (should read like a newspaper headline)

◊ Subtitle (should give basic information about the class or event)

◊ Body—This is where you write a pseudo-news article with the "who, what, where, when and why."

◊ Additional Information

Tip: There are a number of press release templates available online if you search for them. Be sure to choose the one that best reflects your work and will speak to the media outlet where you're sending it.

Write Articles, Essays, and Op-Ed Pieces

Free

More and more, magazines and newspapers are looking for free content to fill their pages. The same is true for blogs and newsletters. If you are a writer, offer to contribute an op-ed piece or a short how-to article in your area of specialty. For example, if you're teaching a class for people with Multiple Sclerosis, pen a short article about the benefits of yoga for someone living with the disease. Various media outlets have different submission guidelines, so it's important to check with them before you send your article.

Some have word-length requirements or require that you publish the article with them exclusively for a given period of time. Some want an email query, others a printed letter. Some want a brief synopsis, while others will want the whole piece. The key is to know how they want their submissions, because not following their guidelines will usually result in your hard work being brushed aside.

Most major newspapers and blogs have submission guidelines on their sites. If they don't, take a moment to call or email, asking how and to whom you should send submissions. While this can be a bit difficult, it's well worth the effort.

Writing an article or essay casts you as an expert in your field. It gives you the opportunity to promote your classes and workshops in subtle, non-pushy ways, and all the while you're drawing on their readers and dramatically increasing your marketing outreach.

It is important to remember that this is not an infomercial. Your article or essay should not read like a sales pitch. The most impressive articles and essays are the ones that are informative and may have little to do with your actual class. They are also the ones that are more likely to get published.

Finally, include a short bio and your website at the end of the piece.

John Smith is a yoga teacher who specializes in working with Multiple Sclerosis and other autoimmune diseases [www.johnsmithyoga.com].

Broadcast Journals

Expensive

Ever wonder how radio and TV producers find all their guests? The vast majority of them are found in trade publications in which potential guests pay to advertise. The downside is that advertising in these journals can be very expensive. The upside is you can get on more shows than you can handle if your ad has the right hook.

When my fourth book, *Hearts and Minds: Talking to Christians about Homosexuality*, came out, my publisher ran an ad in one of the trade publications that simply said, "Interview the author who claims Jesus would embrace homosexuals." My publicist's phone rang off the hook. Of course the topic was both controversial and timely, which helped a lot, but even ads for yoga have yielded substantial results when I provided the proper hook.

While there are many broadcast trade publications, I have found the most widely distributed journal is *Radio-TV Interview Report* (RTIR). The journal offers a print edition and a searchable website for producers and editors [www.RTIR.com].

Appear on TV & Radio

Free/Moderate/Expensive

Appearing as a guest on a radio or TV show is a great way to gain notoriety, but to get bookings, you need to understand how the system works. All producers have one goal in mind—finding topics that speak to and interest their audience. So knowing what audience a given TV or Radio show targets is essential. This is just as true of local media as it is of national media. Producers are not going to invite you on their show to be nice. They're looking for guests who will engage their listeners or viewers and will inspire them to stay tuned in.

For example, NPR's *All Things Considered* is very different from Bill O'Rieley's radio show. The question you need to ask yourself is, "How is my work interesting to the audience of a given show?" That's exactly what the producers of that show are going to be asking.

The best way to get good press is to do something that stands out. Teaching yoga to a unique group of people is one way to do it. Maybe you're teaching a class for wounded soldiers coming back from a war zone, or perhaps you're using yoga as a way to help autistic children. These topics are fresh and interesting and are the types of stories where listeners and viewers can easily become engaged.

Another thing to consider is how you can engage with the audience. Personal stories, facts about your work, relevant statistics, and light banter should all be considered long before you go on the air. It's also advisable to listen to or watch the host interview other guests. Some hosts, like Bill O'Rieley have a very combative approach, whereas Oprah Winfrey has a more conversational approach. Knowing this beforehand is a great way to prepare yourself for the interview.

In addition, if you know something about the host, you can weave something personal about them into the interview. For example, if you are being interviewed about your work with soldiers returning from battle, and you know the host's son is serving in a war zone, you could simply say something like, "I'm sure you son has told you stories about being in the line of fire. Given what researchers have discovered about the harmful effects of stress on both the body and mind, there is perhaps no group of people in America that needs practices like yoga and meditation more than our troops." In doing this you have engaged the host in something that is very personal to him and also explained why the work you are doing is so important.

Five Tips for a Successful Interview

◊ Submit some questions in advance. Not all hosts will use them, but many will—even if they don't, it will force you to think about the questions that will be asked and how you can clearly answer without fumbling for the right words.

◊ Remember the host's name and use it often. The same is true for callers and guests in the audience.

◊ Come with five or six talking points that you want to cover. These talking points should be short bullet points that fit on an index card. Ten pages of notes will do you no good, so keep it very short and sweet. For each talking point, plan a short story that will help the audience connect with the point on an emotional level. The best way to do this is by sharing either a funny or a heartfelt story about a student who benefited from your class, but be sure to maintain confidentiality.

◊ Know your facts. There is nothing worse than being on live TV or radio and being caught unprepared. For example, if you work with autistic children, you should be up on the current research, and never make claims that you can't substantiate. Keep in mind that the host or even a member of the audience might feel the need to correct you, which can be very embarrassing!

◊ Be sure to mention your website at least once during the interview. Better yet, ask the host to say it for you.

Publicists

Expensive

Many of the above marketing tips are used every day by professional publicists. Hiring a publicist can be very, very costly, but if you find the right one, the payoff can be worth it. Even though they will often be doing things that you can do on your own, a good publicist will have something that you won't—connections. They know who to call and frequently have relationships with producers, editors, and journalists. For most yoga teachers, a publicist may be overkill, and well outside their budget. But for teachers who really want to promote their work on the national or international level, working with a professional publicist can be the key that unlocks many important doors and takes your teaching to the next level.

All publicity is good, except an obituary notice.—Brendan Behan

CHAPTER 12:
WEB DESIGN FOR TEACHERS

Looking at the proliferation of personal web pages on the Net, it looks
like very soon everyone on Earth will have 15 megabytes of fame.
—*M.G. Sriram*

As I began the research phase of this book, I started by surveying a number of yoga teachers. Some had been teaching for many years while others were brand new to the profession. What surprised me the most was how many teachers don't have websites. They rely on a Facebook page or the website of the studio at which they teach, but they don't have an online place to call home.

In a sense, I can understand why. The whole process of posting and maintaining a website can feel daunting—especially if you are not tech savvy. Yet, bowing to this fear puts you at a significant disadvantage. A website today is every bit as important as a business card was in years past.

In this chapter, I will be going over some basic concepts to help you get started. However, one chapter is not enough to teach you everything there is to know about web design. If that is your goal, you will probably need some schooling. My goal is to help you understand some of the basics so you can approach a web designer in an organized and informed fashion.

Working with a Web Designer

Web designers, at least the good ones, are wildly creative people. Think of them as interior designers for your online life. Yet like an interior designer, they need your input. Their job is not to design a website that reflects their own tastes. Their job is to build a site that represents you and your work. They will guide the process, but approaching them with some sort of a vision for what you want is key.

Aside from owning a piece of internet real estate that accurately reflects you, it's important to remember that designers charge by the hour. If you come to them with nothing in hand, you will wind up spending a lot more for your website. If you take the time to map out your site, provide them with quality photos, and have your text written in advance, the process will run much more smoothly, and the invoice you receive from them in the end will not break the bank.

Web Hosts and Domain Names

Your website will need to live on a server somewhere. A server is a huge computer that hosts thousands of other websites and provides basic services, such as email, statistics on who is visiting your site, and what sites they're coming from. This is important because you can see if your marketing efforts with services like *Google Ad Words* are paying off.

Most web hosting services also enable you to host a database, run blogging software like Word Press, set up forms, and use shopping carts. Each service is a bit different, so you need to examine the features offered at a few companies to make sure they offer the features you want without paying for a lot of stuff you don't need. Generally speaking, a yoga teacher's website should cost less than twenty dollars (U.S.) per month. This cost will go up if your traffic increases dramatically, but in the beginning that should not be a problem.

Your domain name is a separate but related issue. When you type in my URL, www.darrenmain.com, your computer quickly checks with the computer gods and finds out where to direct you. Regardless of where you are in the world, if you type in that URL, you will get to my website. Yet, this does not happen because a magic leprechaun guided your web browser to the proper place. It happened because I paid for and registered my URL.

Most web hosting services will do this for you, but you can save yourself a lot of time if you make a list of five or six URLs that you would like to have. Once you start the registration process, you will be offered the opportunity to lease your desired name. Although you will likely do the whole process through your web host, you are paying for two separate services—the monthly fee your web host charges you to have your site live on their server and a yearly lease for your domain name.

Tip: Once you register your domain name, even if you use your web host to do it, that name is yours for the length of time you maintain the lease. Should you decide to switch the company that hosts your site, your domain name will follow you.

Once you set up your web hosting with a given company, they will send you an email. This email is very important, as it will have the codes necessary to upload and edit your site. They will also give you a link to your dashboard where you can set up your email accounts, check statistics, and do all sorts of other useful things.

Ingredients

Text

Your website is going to need text. Unless you plan to hire a professional writer, you will need to write that text yourself. As a general rule, you can provide your web designer with a page–by–page list of the text you want to include. Things like your teacher bio, descriptions of your classes, the addresses of the studios where you teach, and so on, all need to be authored by you, and preferably before you meet with your web designer for the first time.

Photos

The old adage is true—a picture tells a thousand words. The question is what will those thousand words tell visitors to your site about you. If you have your friend take photos of you with her camera phone, you will be telling the visitors to your site a lot—mostly that you are not a professional.

One of the most important things you can do is invest in good photos taken by a professional who knows a thing or two about good lighting. Photo editing can only take a bad photo so far. It's also important to consider the tones and colors you want to use on your site. If your site has a lot of earth tones, you may want to post photos in sepia tone. If your site is bright and sunny, you may want to use color photos featuring you and your models wearing colors that blend with your site. And if your site has an artistic feel, you may want to use black and white images. A good photographer can help you choose colors and tones that will convey the message and theme of your site.

Photos posted to your site will need to be of a lower resolution than the ones you use for printed material; however, your web designer can easily adjust the size of the images if you provide files that are larger. It is always better to provide high-resolution photos as they can easily be scaled down, but you can't make them larger without making them fuzzy. Photos posted to your website will need to be in jpeg format, but again, your designer can convert them to jpeg if necessary.

Graphics

Photos are not the only images on your website. Most websites have a variety of other images, such as title bars and menus. Generally speaking, your web designer will create these images for you, but if you provide them yourself, they need to be in gif format.

Audio

Some websites use audio. For example, you may want your website to play some new-age music. I generally steer people away from this, as many people find musical web sites annoying—especially if they are surfing the web at work rather than being productive—at least from their boss' point of view. In any event, if you decide to have audio on your site, you will need to provide the audio to your web designer in mp3 format. If the file is music, you will want to make sure the bit rate is set to at least 128 bps. If however, you are doing spoken word, such as posting a talk you give on the benefits of inversions, then you can use a much lower bit rate.

Video

Currently, we are seeing more and more video footage on the internet. There was a time when Adobe Flash was your only option for having video on your site. With the advent of HTML-5, the latest standard for websites, there are more options available. If you want video on your site, make sure you know a thing or two about filming and editing a quality video. You may want to hire a professional to produce your video for you. Otherwise, your video will look more like grainy porn from the 70's, rather than video that will inspire people to attend your classes. Most web designers will ask you to provide video files in mpeg format.

Hyper Links

The thing that makes the World Wide Web a "web" is hyperlinks. Your site may be its own domain, but it is intimately connected with countless other sites via hyperlinks. In your professional bio, for example, you may want to link to the teachers with whom you have studied. You may want to have a resource page that links to your favorite yoga studios, or you may want to link to a Google map so people can easily find your studio.

Whatever links you want to include should be submitted to your web designer with the text. Be sure to include the full link including the http://. This will insure your links actually work.

Embedded Code

Websites like YouTube and Amazon now offer you the ability to embed code into your website; this allows your visitors to interact with the content without leaving your site. For example, if you want to post a video from YouTube to your site, you can get the HTML code from the YouTube site and paste it into the HTML code of your site. Then when people visit your site they can play the video right there.

This may sound difficult, but it's actually quite easy. Your web designer can guide you further. If you're not sure how to pull the code from a given site, simply give the web designer the URL of the content you would like to embed and he/she can advise you.

Sample HTML Code

<iframe title="YouTube video player" width="640" height="390" src="http://www.youtube.com/embed/2h-6ZqCi-Tg" frameborder="0" allowfullscreen></iframe>

Metta Tags

By providing a list of key words, search engines can better catalog your site. Your designer will know what to do with the list, but you will move the process along more efficiently if you provide them with a list separated by commas, which they can then embed into the code of your site.

Site Mapping

A site map is a visual representation of your site that is sketched out. It doesn't need to be fancy, but it is very important. Each page should be represented, and you can draw lines to each page showing how you want the site to link together.

The site map will be an important tool for your web designer, and it will also help you organize your thoughts and gather together the text, links, photos, and other elements that your designer will need when pulling your site together.

Following are a few pages you will want to consider including in your site map:

Home Page

The home page is the first page people see when they go to your URL. The big mistake people make with their home page is putting in too much information. Like the cover of a magazine, it should provide an overview of the site and easy access to the content you have posted on other pages. The home page is always named index.html.

Teacher Bio

Your bio page is a place where people can learn a bit more about you, both professionally and personally. It typically includes one paragraph about where you studied and with whom, followed by a second paragraph talking about the style or styles of yoga you teach.

Schedule

Your schedule page can provide a list of the classes you teach, as well as locations, times, and styles. This is a great page to link to a Google map for each class. If the studio where you teach offers online registration for your class, you can provide a link to that page on their website as well.

Resources

A resource page is a great place for students to find things that will augment their practice. Some resources may include yoga related websites, teachers with whom you have studied, books, music, and even other healing professionals in your community. If you are going to link to books and music, it's a good idea to set up an affiliate account with a company like Amazon so you will get a small stipend for the referral. You may not make a lot of money, but it could be enough to offset the cost of hosting your site.

Blog

Your blog is a great pace to post updates, yoga related articles, videos from YouTube, and other tidbits that will keep your students returning to your site. Setting up a blog is not easy and you will probably need the help of your web designer, but it is well worth the effort!

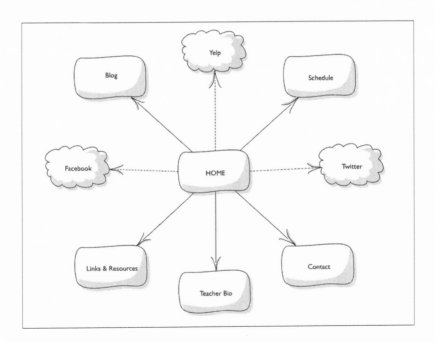

Design Tips

When I was going through my drug use phase, my father and mother learned that I was unsuccessfully trying to grow pot in my bedroom. Being conservative, they flew off the deep end. My stints with drinking were upsetting to them, but pot was a 'real drug' in their minds.

So I decided to calm them down by using my stoner logic. "If pot is so bad, how come it is illegal to drink and drive and not illegal to smoke pot and drive?" I reasoned. I'm not sure why people who are stoned think they deserve to be made captain of the debate team, but that was a delusion that seemed to grow deeper with every bong hit for me.

Needless to say, my father's Vulcan logic silenced me. "First, that is not true. Second, there is a saying, *Just because you can, doesn't mean you should.*"

I don't remember much from that time in my life, although I could probably still roll a joint blindfolded if need be. But for some reason, that simple bit of logic stuck in my head, and nowhere has that notion served me better than in design.

Websites can be built with an endless variety of colors, fonts, text styles, animated graphics, roll over links, sounds, videos, and text treatments. As you design your site, whether you use a web designer or go it alone, always remember—Just because you can, doesn't mean you should!

Text

If you think back over the last twenty websites you visited, you probably didn't do much scrolling. We live in a sound bite world, and nowhere is that more evident than on the internet. People simply don't read more than a few paragraphs at a time. It's okay to have multiple web pages, but if the average person needs to scroll, they will probably get bored and go to another website. When it comes to text—Just because you can, doesn't mean you should!

Color

Just because you have a virtual crayon box at your disposal doesn't mean you should use every crayon. Websites that look like a Christmas tree with flashing colored lights are a tacky eyesore and come off as very unprofessional. Rather than use twenty colors, use two or three that complement the mood and tone you are trying to create. When it comes to color—Just because you can, doesn't mean you should!

Font

There was a time when almost all websites used the New Times Roman font. Today there are more web friendly fonts available, and with the HTML-5 as the new standard, font choices will increase again. The good news is that this gives designers a lot more flexibility. The bad news is that not all fonts look good on a computer screen and many can strain the eyes.

There are two basic font styles—Serif and Sans Serif. Basically a Serif font has a finishing stroke attached to each letter, whereas a Sans Serif font does not. Some people believe Serif fonts are easier to read while others argue that Sans Serif fonts are easier. And by argue, I mean just that—typesetters have very strong feelings about this issue in much the same way editors may not agree about when to use an em-dash (long hyphen) and when to use a comma or semicolon. Regardless of your point of view on this issue, following are the important things to know about choosing fonts:

◊ Never use more than three fonts on a page (or website). Many would argue that two is the limit.

◊ It is best to use all Sans Serif or all Serif fonts. In other words, don't mix New Times Roman with Arial.

◊ While fancy fonts may be a lot of fun, they are horrible on the eyes. In the battle between fancy verses legible, you should always side with the legible fonts!

◊ When it comes to fonts—Just because you can, doesn't mean you should!

Professional Graphics and Photos

As we have already discussed, photos and graphics will set a tone for your site at least as much if not more than the text itself. You should really consider what image you are going to post to your site. For example, on my website I have chosen to use photos that depict happy people doing yoga with me assisting them. This was a very conscious choice because I wanted people visiting my site to see a visual representation of what I try to create in my class. This may not be the look and feel you are going for, but whatever you decide, make it a conscious choice.

Tips for Graphics and Photos

◊ Unless you are a graphic designer or you are married to a professional photographer, pay someone!

◊ Not every space on a website needs to be filled with an image or text. White space is good! One well-placed image will likely be more effective than twenty images.

◊ It is bad karma to use a photo or image without getting permission from the photographer or designer. Some will want money; others may be happy to share their work with you in exchange for proper credit.

◊ If you don't want to hire a photographer, you can easily buy stock photos depicting various yoga poses through a number of websites such as www.istockphoto.com

◊ When it comes to photos and images—Just because you can, doesn't mean you should!

Paragraph Centering

What the mullet did for hair, centering text did to design. Just as you would not send your child out of the house with a mullet, you should not put your website up with lots of centered text. A title here or a quote set apart from the main body of the text is one thing, but to center every word on your page is a nightmare to read and it screams unprofessional! When it comes to centering—Just because you can, doesn't mean you should!

Do It Yourself

If you are a bit tech savvy, and you want to try designing your own site, there are a few resources that will help you along the way. Web design software has made creating a professional-looking site easier these days, and there are a few books out there that can help you as well.

Recommended Reading

Web Design for Dummies by Lisa Lopuck

Learning Web Design: A Beginner's Guide to HTML, Graphics, and Beyond by Jennifer Niederst Robbins

Software

Adobe Dreamweaver (OS X /Windows) www.adobe.com

Sandvox (OS X) www.karelia.com

WeBuilder (Windows) www.blumentals.net

CONCLUSION

About a year after I moved to San Francisco, my father called and asked me to come to the family pig roast. This annual event is attended by hundreds of our friends and relatives from around the country. At the time, I was a bit of a black sheep in the family. Being the only vegetarian at a pig roast is a bit like showing up drunk at an AA meeting. People were generally glad to see me there, but I could see the concern in their eyes.

In addition to not eating meat, I lived in San Francisco—which one of my more crude uncles referred to as, "The land of fruits and nuts." The news of my coming out of the closet had spread through the family tree like beech bark disease, and to top it off, I was a yoga teacher. With the exception of a few uncles, my family has always accepted my unconventional ways, and has, for the most part, treated me with respect in spite of my quirkiness.

So I made my way from cousin to cousin, from aunt to uncle, and on to people I didn't even know. As with any occasion where small talk is all you have time for, the subject of my occupation inevitably came up.

The responses were as varied as they were amusing.

"So you're a Hindu?"

"So you're a Buddhist?"

"Can you put your foot behind your head?"

And a litany of other questions that are not appropriate for mixed company.

A few years later, I went to another family reunion and, again the subject of my occupation repeatedly came up. Yet in a few short years, the questions were notably different.

"Why do they call it downward dog?"

"I have thought about taking yoga, but I'm not flexible enough."

"I heard Oprah does yoga; have your ever met her?"

This past summer I returned once again to the pig roast, and yet again I was peppered with questions about my work.

"My doctor told me I should eat more vegetarian food. Do you have any advice?"

"I've been thinking about doing yoga for my bad back. How do I get started?"

"What style of yoga would be best to lower my blood pressure?"

"Will you teach me to meditate?"

Rather than being the black sheep, my chosen profession was a topic of genuine interest by people who, a few years earlier, viewed it as, in the words of the same, crude uncle, an activity reserved for "hippies, homos, and Hindus." (The fact that I embodied two out of three of his ignorant stereotypes only seemed to narrow his mind further.) Like the doctor who goes to the family gathering only to be questioned about strange skin disorders while she is trying to eat her potato salad, I was getting questions from every angle. Gone were the days when I was the black sheep; now people who had once scoffed at my crazy ways seemed excited to learn more and were even considering some lifestyle changes.

There has never been a better time, at least here in the west, for people to practice and teach yoga. Yoga has the support of doctors, chiropractors, psychotherapists, and even some religious leaders. Its benefits have been demonstrated over and over in peer-reviewed scientific literature, and more than a million people practice it in some form every day in the United States alone.

The profession of teaching yoga has gained a tremendous amount of respect by the population at large with people of every stripe—young and old, rich and poor, Christian, Jewish and atheist. Its reach has moved deep into the White, Latino, Asian, and African American communities, and better yet, people of every race, religion, and sexual orientation are practicing together in harmony.

Yet, with all this good news, many yoga teachers fail to see that we can no longer teach as though we are born black sheep. We need to be true to yoga and the principles that guide this ancient practice, while presenting it to the world in a way that invites and welcomes the diverse populations that are hungry for the physical, emotional, psychological, and spiritual healing that yoga offers.

To do this, we must treat our teaching like an ethical business—one that is rooted deeply in the yamas and niyamas, and one that meets potential students where they are, rather than where we think they should be. When we run our teaching like an ethical business, we open ourselves up to more and more students. When we run our teaching like an ethical business, other healing professionals will continue to value what we do and will work in tandem with us.

Certainly this book doesn't hold all the answers, but I do hope it will help you to reach more students, to work more effectively with other professionals, and to support you in your efforts to move yoga forward.

We stand at a great crossroads as teachers. Either we act in haphazard and unethical ways, ignoring the principles that have guided yoga for millennia, or we step up and recognize that although yoga is changing on the surface, the bedrock of our practice remains the same. There is nothing in the ancient texts that declares we need to starve in order to be true yogis, but much is written about acting from a moral and ethical place.

By returning to our roots, we can take a huge step forward as individual teachers and as a community. The day is coming when all of us will attend family gatherings, church potlucks, and other social events where we will be held in very high esteem—not because we are special, but because the magic of yoga will have spread to every corner of western culture.

By following your dharma, you will help to bring yoga to hundreds or thousands of people who have been waiting for your unique voice, your unique teaching style, and the unique energy and passion that you bring to the yoga mat. In order to do this most effectively, however, you will need to devote your life to the profession of teaching. It is not enough to show up and teach. Your yoga needs to reach into your continuing education, your accounting, and your marketing. It needs to touch your professional ethics and inspire the creative ways in which you offer yoga through classes, workshops, and retreats.

I define yoga as *the bringing together of that which is <u>perceived</u> to be separate.* The time has come for yoga teachers to recognize that yoga happens as much when you balance your checkbook as it does when you sit in meditation. There can be as much yoga in marketing as there is in sitting in full lotus. All the elements of being a yogi entrepreneur are one in truth, and the sadhana (practice) of the yoga teacher is to recognize that unity. Once we realize this, our business will flourish, and our students will find the healing and spiritual fulfillment they are seeking.

Appendix

Resources

Professional Organizations

The Yoga Alliance • www.yogaalliance.org

Suppliers

Hugger Mugger • www.huggermugger.com

Yoga Props • www.yogaprops.net

Lululemon • www.lululemon.com

Giam • www.gaiam.com

Accounting and Insurance

Yoga Journal Yoga Teacher Liability Insurance
  • www.yogajournal.com/for_teachers

Mindbody Software • www.mindbodyonline.com

Yoga Magazines & Websites

Yoga Journal • www.yogajournal.com

Yoga International • www.himalayaninstitute.org/yi/

Yoga Magazine • www.yogamagazine.co.uk

Online Printers

Overnight Prints • www.overnightprints.com

Remembering Arthur Leiper

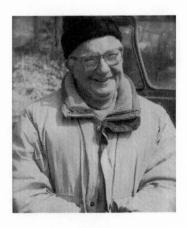

Somewhere in India, November 2009

In so many ways I have been blessed with a wonderful and supportive family. Both in terms of material needs as well as emotional support, my family, though not without faults, is top notch. In fact, the only thing that I was denied with regard to family was grandparents, as all four of them had passed away before my first birthday.

There are many things that parents can teach their children, but there are some things that only a family member who is a generation removed can offer. They have a wisdom that can only be garnered by many years of experience and even at a young age, I knew that for all the blessings my family had to bestow, I still felt cheated by not having even one grandparent to whom I could turn. It was not until I met Arthur Leiper that I knew what it felt like to have a grandfather.

When I was in the sixth grade, I was forced to repeat a year of school and this resulted in my also having to repeat a year of CCD, the Roman Catholic equivalent of Sunday school. A curse, or so it seemed. In many ways that was one of the hardest years of my young life. The loss of friends, feelings of failure, and the belief that I was stupid all contributed to a number of self-destructive behaviors. But I believe that no pain or hardship is placed at our feet without the support to overcome that challenge. I didn't learn much about Jesus, the Bible, or the sacraments in CCD, but I was given two invaluable pearls of wisdom that were far more important.

The first was that the angels God sends to us in times of need are not always cloaked in white robes. In fact, most often they are ordinary people who stop long enough to take notice when you are in need. This was the case when I met Arthur Leiper, my CCD teacher. For whatever reason, he saw something in me that few others could. He took a liking to me and always seemed to see my potential even when I couldn't see it in myself.

When I was in school for social work, I read a study in which highly successful and well adjusted adults who had experienced extreme abuse as children were surveyed. The researchers were trying to find out what these people had in common that allowed them to transcend the brutality of their pasts when so few others are able to. Although all of their stories were quite different, they all had one very important thing in common. All of them could identify at least one adult in their childhood who believed in them and who looked out for them. That adult, be it a family member, teacher, priest or rabbi, was an anchor of sorts and allowed the child to weather the storm and ultimately flourish as an adult. Although my childhood was not traumatic when compared to the experiences of many, Arthur Leiper was my anchor during one of the most difficult times in my life.

Arthur also taught me my first mantra. Typically, a mantra is a sacred word in an ancient language that is repeated over and over to keep guiding the mind back to its spiritual center. His mantra was far more simple than that, however. It didn't matter what Christian principle he was trying to teach. He always reminded us that to practice the teaching of Jesus was difficult because it was not in our nature to do so. Over and over again he would say, "It goes against the grain!" Whether turning the other cheek, caring for the needy, practicing forgiveness, or putting the needs of others ahead of our own selfish desires, he always reminded us that to do these things was often challenging, but that we had the power to choose. Over the years, when I have found myself in moral quandaries or struggling to be a compassionate and mindful yoga teacher, Art's mantra has echoed in my head.

A few months ago, Arthur learned that he had Leukemia. Unfortunately none of the available treatments were effective and he passed away earlier this week. I learned the news via an email from my sister-in-law while still in Rishikesh, India. At first I was in shock and being so far away from my family, I was having trouble finding a way to honor his passing. Had

I been in the USA, I would certainly have attended a Catholic Mass, but since Catholic churches are rare in India, I felt like a tiny boat lost at sea. I wasn't sure how to grieve.

Arthur was more than just a CCD teacher to me. After the school year ended, we maintained a friendship. It was Arthur who taught me to navigate the subway system in Boston and ultimately became my sponsor when I received the Catholic sacrament of Confirmation. One summer, while I was a camp counselor in Maine, he and my brother drove up to surprise me and arrived on the day I was feeling most homesick.

Art gave me my first lessons in public speaking, loaned me the money for my first yoga teacher training, and came to visit me while I was at the ashram so I would not be alone for Thanksgiving. He even managed to bring my father along for the ride, which was nothing short of a miracle. Although he didn't always understand my ways, he never failed to support me. It didn't matter that I was a yoga teacher rather than a Catholic priest, or that I dated boys instead of girls. It didn't matter to him that I lived on the West coast and rarely got to see him. He was always there with his characteristic crooked smile, and quirky laugh.

His friendship extended to the rest of my family as well, and he was very supportive of my parents when they divorced. In recent years he and his wife Mary regularly joined our family for holiday meals.

In addition to his family, Art loved two things in this world. The first was his Catholic faith; the second was trains. He loved to take trains anywhere and everywhere. He built model trains by hand and had many of the Amtrak lines and schedules committed to memory.

Given that I felt so removed from my family, and I couldn't find a Catholic church where I could honor him, I felt as though I were letting him down. But fate has an interesting way of giving us what we need. As I write this I'm on a train chugging through India with tears pouring down my face. It doesn't seem to matter that I'm surrounded by a bunch of Indians who clearly think I have lost my mind, because this is the perfect place to reflect on the blessing of having known Arthur Lieper.

It is because of him that I am here today—that I get to travel to far-off countries and to teach yoga. It is because of him that I was able to find my way around the very congested Haridwar train station this morning and it is because of him that I occasionally make the right choices in life, even when "it goes against the grain" to do so.

Life won't be the same without Arthur, but I do know that he will be with me each time I ride a train or reflect on the true meaning of family. I hope and pray that I can follow his example and rise above my ego long enough to see the potential in a stranger, even when they are struggling to see it in themselves. Thank you Arthur for being the grandfather I never had, the angel I most needed, and a life long friend. I will miss you deeply.

ACKNOWLEDGEMENTS

Special thanks to my family:

My son Jaden, my mother Kathy Ascare, my father John Main, my brother Jason Main, and my sister Jennifer Main-Holdridge, my nieces Zoe Main, Haley Holdridge, and Lauren Glaza, and my nephews, Chase, Jake, and Tyler Flynn. Also to the Mains and Flynns: Don, Amy, Alden, Josie, Joe, John, Sarah, Peter, Linda, Kate, Gus and Adelina.

To all the People who have supported Jaden and helped bring him safely into my home and my heart. . . .

Amirah Salaam, Abby Williams, and the entire team at Family Builders, Rodney Marlin, Kaaren Alvarado, Krisztina Abonyi Bernstein at Conductiva, Barbara Bratton, Jennifer Daly, Dr. Hannah Glass, Suzanne Golden and her team, Zoe Levitt, Dr. Sue Rhee, Dr. Marie Ribeiro and countless others who cared for Jaden before he came to me and who continue to support him in his healing.

Special thanks to the many friends who have supported me so much:

Jim Healy & Patrick Meyer, Lance King, Michael Lynch, Christopher Love, Jasper Trout, Craig Daniel, Michael Watson, Sue Louiseau, Kevin Hicks, Wanda Pierce, Tim and Tara Dale, Kimberly Wilson, Michael Alexander, Sam Jackson, Jamie Lindsay, Christine Maggiore, Robin Scovill, Ryan Brewer and Bodhi Maisha, Rodney Marlin, Amirah Salaam, Abby Williams, Adair Sapinski, Jack Mueller, Ellie Brown, Yogi Amrit Desai, Kamini Desai

To my editors:

Sue Louiseau and Peter Wong—Thank you so much for your tireless efforts in editing my words in this book and in everything I write. You both have the patience of a saint to be able to deal with my spelling!

I would also like to thank my entire editing team:

Sylvie Anne Williams, Tiffany Hualin Raether, Maria Christina, Jeremi McManus, Christopher Love, Liz Filippone, and Michael Fantasia.

Special thanks to Jasper Trout for creating such a beautiful cover for this book.

Made in the USA
Lexington, KY
07 June 2013